MW01235734

The Sleep Guide of Your Dreams

Strategies and Habits for a Smarter Sleep to Enhance Performance, Health, and Happiness

BLAKE HAYNES

Disclaimer Notice:

Please note the information contained within this document is for educational and entertainment purposes only. All effort has been executed to present accurate, up to date, and reliable, complete information. No warranties of any kind are declared or implied. Readers acknowledge that the author is not engaging in the rendering of legal, financial, medical or professional advice. The content within this book has been derived from various sources. Please consult a licensed professional before attempting any techniques outlined in this book.

By reading this document, the reader agrees that under no circumstances is the author responsible for any losses, direct or indirect, which are incurred as a result of the use of the information contained within this document, including, but not limited to, — errors, omissions, or inaccuracies.

Table of Contents

Chapter 9 : Goodbye Jetlag! 150

Chapter 10: Now What? 161

Conclusion... 167

Resources 174

Introduction

The human brain is the most resilient and sophisticated biological complex known to man. With virtually no limits to its processing power and storage, the human brain is built to control the human body for as long as we live. However, even the brain and body need to recharge from time to time, and sleep is the only true way by which our body, mind, and brain recoup lost vitality and keep us in perfect shape to maximize our potentials. Unfortunately, we have never had it this bad with sleep!

Life on Planet Earth is at a frenetic pace that has not been seen before, and we need more and better sleep now more than ever. Unfortunately, and for entirely avoidable reasons, advancements in digital technology mean that the lines between work and home are continuously blurred and eroded, and an increasing number of people are being deprived of good quality sleep. As a race, the CDC says we are at 'epidemic level' when it comes to getting adequate rest and sleep, and the worst part of it all is that most sufferers do not even know.

The facts about average sleeping habits paint a grim picture.

o In the United States, 35% of people do not get up to seven hours of sleep each night

o About 50-70 million Americans have a full-blown sleeping disorder

o Between 1985 and now, the percentage of people that sleep for less than seven hours has increased significantly by 31%

o Worldwide, 10% of adults are battling with chronic insomnia

o Sleep deprivation costs the United States 411 billion dollars in economic loss yearly

o 21% of women suffer from obstructive apnea while as high as 31% of the male population deal with the same issue

If that does not immediately set the alarm bells tolling, consider the effects of not sleeping well or long enough.

Mentally, sleep is essentially a chance to reset your mind and body to their default state daily. So, when you do not get enough sleep, you carry your problems over to the next day. That means you are forever bogged down mentally. The resultant stress can leave you feeling irritable or sensitive. That can lead to avoidable arguments, panic attacks, angry outbursts, relationship problems, loss of focus, and rash decisions.

Reduced sleep quality puts your body through physiological stress that it is not designed to withstand for long. You are not a robot – your body needs rest to function optimally. Therefore, it is no surprise that chronic lack of sleep leaves you susceptible to immune dysfunction and conditions such as heart attacks, strokes, diabetes, obesity, and hypertension. To buttress this, a 2013 study reported that people who sleep for less than six hours daily have a 32% increased chance of developing hypertension. Virtually every single system is affected when you deprive yourself of sleep constantly. In fact, sleep insufficiency is a health condition itself and deserves all the attention it can get.

As I am sure you know, it is no news that sleeping problems can affect performance, cause work accidents, and account for a large drop in productivity. With sleep loss comes a loss of vigor, vitality, and concentration. This has resulted in a lot of morbidities and casualties. For instance, a study conducted in 2014 reported that drivers with poor quality of sleep are 3.35 times as likely to be involved in a road accident than drivers that got at least 8 hours of sleep. When you align this finding with the fact that drowsy driving has been fingered as the cause of 1,550 deaths and 40,000 injuries annually in the United States, sleep deprivation certainly becomes a major issue. If that is not scary, I don't know what is.

The good news is **there is a fix for your sleep problems.** We have been gifted the chance to control our sleep routines, but most people abuse sleep through habits that interfere significantly with the ideal sleep patterns. Hectic work schedules, physical exertions, relationship problems, mental breakdowns, and emotional dysregulation all contribute to incredible levels of stress that can affect one's sleep. For most people, they simply borrow from time reserved for sleeping to complete their daily tasks, with no intention or means of repaying. Throw in negative lifestyle and nutritional choices, and you have a potent mix that can disrupt the body's normal inclination and ability to recharge itself through sleep.

Do you have trouble switching off that nagging voice in your head at night? Do you wake up each morning feeling foggy, heavy, and unrefreshed? Do you spend countless hours trying to get some shuteye?

If you have answered in the affirmative to any of the questions above, then, I have written this book **for you**. I know the facts I have quoted sound *scary,* but the power to restore your sleep to its default pattern is in your hands right now. Human beings are the only mammals who are able to delay sleep willingly. That knowledge is the key to resolving your sleep problems. By being intentional about your sleeping habits and learning how to optimize your nighttime routine, you can turn this around and relearn how to sleep better and for longer.

As a performance strategist, I have over a decade of experience helping hundreds of individuals optimize their daily lives for peak performance, health, and happiness. At the beginning of my career, most of my efforts with my clients were directed at implementing the right nutrition, exercise, and stress management protocols. Like most therapists and strategists, sleep represented only a small, grossly-overlooked, fraction of the equation. I was guilty of this too until I had a particularly rough time and experienced the firsthand, devastating consequences of inadequate sleep over a few months.

In just over twelve weeks, I had changed almost completely. I was near burnout, prone to anger, more sensitive, always exhausted, easily hurt, and notably, my performance at work dropped. I missed appointments and forgot tasks; I gradually lost interest in work, and going home became a mood-sapping event too. Then, it hit me! My inability to sleep had been at the root cause of the changes in my life – this experience served as a powerful epiphany that led me to dive into the cutting-edge science on the topic of sleep. I distilled the content I found into practical, actionable steps that I could put in place to get my clients the top results they were looking for. The result of optimizing their sleep had an unparalleled impact on their overall wellbeing, productivity, and health.

I have written this book to make these strategies available to the general population in the hopes of making the widely spread sleep crisis less so. Built upon my experience, strategies, and the most recent scientific evidence, consider this a manual and guide for changing your sleeping patterns and enjoying the renewed vitality that comes with sleeping the right way.

Adequate sleep confers you with a lot of personal, interpersonal, performance, and health advantages. These advantages include adequate ability to deal with stress, improved relationships and reduced risk for conditions such as depression, strokes, cancers, and diabetes. Other advantages include significant control over your moods, optimal metabolism, improved ability to focus on tasks, a better productivity ratio, a sharper, short- and long-term memory and improved resistance to diseases. I know this because I have overseen these improvements (in business, emotional intelligence, overall performance, health, and relationships) in hundreds of clients who have implemented the strategies in this book.

I remember one client in particular, let's call him David for the sake of anonymity, whose situation I am sure you'll be able to relate to on some level. He was in his mid-thirties at the time, a serial entrepreneur who was devoted to providing the best material comforts for his two children and wife Sarah. In trying to juggle multiple businesses, family life, and his personal life, he started to sacrifice sleep. Like most people, he needed more time for his tasks and obligations, and he simply continued to borrow from the time allocated for sleep. Daily, he stayed up late, drank multiple cups of coffee and shot out of bed even before the alarm went off, in a bid to do as much work as possible. He became so used to this lifestyle that he could not even sleep without a bottle or two of alcohol.

Over time, his performance at work began to suffer – he picked quarrels easily and disrupted team performance. It was almost as if the harder he worked, the lesser the benefits he reaped. He did not find satisfaction in family life either – he was moody and insensitive to the emotional needs of his partner. He knew something had to change. So, he came to me. It didn't take much time to notice the telltale signs of sleep deprivation. We started working together with a large focus on his sleep hygiene, and almost immediately, he noticed an impact on his productivity, mood, and general. The strategies that saved his work and marriage are the exact ones I'll be unveiling in this book.

Do you sense a kindred spirit in David? Are you going through a similar phase and in need of relief? Do you have unresolved problems with your relationships and work? Have you been trying to boost your productivity with no success?

My promise to you is that you will have all the knowledge and practical tools necessary to take your sleep to the next level and reap the rewards in return. In exchange, you must promise not to overlook any sentence or aspect of this book. Every chapter and paragraph is built to dovetail into the next while helping you to build a new routine that will optimize your sleep.

Have you ever told yourself, "I'll have a late one tonight; I can simply catch up on sleep this weekend."? I am sorry to burst that bubble, but scientific proof says you need to sleep for more hours than you have missed, to get any semblance of recovery. That means it is not mathematically feasible for you to repay your sleep debt since most people owe some sleep every weeknight. The debt just continues to grow to staggering levels. With this in mind, it is even more important to get adequate sleep every day. You simply cannot afford to wait – the earlier you can get better sleep, the better it is for you.

This book contains strategies guaranteed to turn your life around drastically if implemented completely and correctly. You will learn how nutrition, light, space, work, and your moods affect your sleep. I will show you how to get in sync with your body's internal clock, discover powerful stress-relieving techniques, develop your bedtime ritual, create a sleep sanctuary and fully regulate your circadian rhythm to get the best possible sleep you can. Most importantly, you need to begin to act on the tips and strategies. It is vital for you and your health – and you need to start now!

Good luck!

Chapter 1: Why You Need Sleep

Our brain and body work every second of every day to keep us alive and in a position where we can maximize our potential. However, it is not feasible to expect our brain to work at the same intensity for the whole of the day. Sleep, therefore, is a chance for the brain to rest a bit and process the plethora of data you have loaded onto it during the day. This need has directed our sleeping routine since we started the evolution journey. Basically, sunrise and sunset dictate when we should stay awake and when we need to get out of bed. Unfortunately, it is not always possible to follow this route. Sleep is easily postponed or shifted back by people in favor of other activities such as seeing a movie or making a long-distance call. That doesn't mean that the quality and quantity of sleep you get does not matter. It does, and as

21

a result, let me ask you a question. "On average, how many hours do you sleep for daily?"

For everyone, the required minimum quantity of sleep should not be less than seven to eight hours. That means you should spend a third of your days sleeping. Do you sleep for as long as that?

I understand that it may be hard for you to give an exact estimate of how long you sleep for daily. So, here are a few more signs that can tell you that you are not getting enough sleep.

Signs That You Are Not Getting Enough Sleep

- **Drowsiness**

Do you doze off during the day, even in the midst of important events? Are you the guy that regularly misses his station because he dozed off on the metro? Do you often find yourself falling asleep in awkward places and at inconvenient times? This is usually a signal that you are not getting enough sleep.

- **Waking Up Unrefreshed**

Do you feel heavy and tired when you wake up? Do you have to spend the first few minutes after waking up to force yourself onto your feet? Do you wake up in the morning feeling exactly the same way you felt before going to bed? That may be an indication that there is a problem with the duration or quality of the sleep you are getting each night.

- **Excessive Consumption Of Caffeine**

I understand that you may like tea a lot, but are you addicted to caffeine? Is coffee your savior from drowsiness each morning? Do you need to get some caffeine into your system to stop all the yawns and keep moving on? If yes, then you may already have sleeping problems.

- **Sudden Weight Gain**

Poor quality of sleep can cause weight gain. I will explore this further in the next section, but gaining weight rapidly without any alternative explanation can be a result of sleep deprivation.

- **Physical Appearance**

Take a look at yourself in the mirror this morning. What do you see? Do you see a bubbling, energetic, and active face staring back at you? Or is it only the eye bags, puffy eyelids, red shot eyes and yawns that you can see? Physical appearance can give away a poor sleeping habit. You just need to know what to look out for.

- **Forgetfulness And Inability To Concentrate**

If you forget facts easily and find it hard to concentrate as much as you should/can, then it may be time to look at your sleeping habit. If you do not sleep enough, you may find it harder to focus during the day until you have napped at least.

The Dangers Of Sleep Deprivation

What happens when you make a habit out of not sleeping long and well enough? Is there any potential damage to your body and mind when you have a poor sleeping habit?

"Yes!" is the answer to both questions. Sleep is the body's choice for catching up on events of the last few hours to keep you fresh for tomorrow. Sleep is intimately tied to several biochemical and metabolic processes that leave little room for sharp changes. Therefore, any potential changes in your routine that can infringe upon the quality and quantity of sleep you get is harmful to your health and performance in the short, mid, and long-term.

Let us take a closer look at some of the potential dangers of sleep deprivation on your physical and mental health.

Sleep And Physical Health
- **Effect On Memory**

Sleeping is the final piece in memory-acquisition – it is a necessary prerequisite for memory consolidation? First, let's start by answering what memory consolidation is.

During the day, the brain continues to stack up information from all sensory organs. Usually, we may not even realize that our brain has picked up some extra information. However, the brain does not immediately process all this information. Rather, when we sleep, the

25

brain proceeds at a leisurely pace to link events, emotions, projections, and gestures together to form whole pictures of what has happened during the day. That is why you can go to bed undecided over a choice you have to make and wake up fully sure of the right decision to make. It's because you have allowed your brain a chance to look at all the variables and connect them together.

When it comes to knowledge acquisition, the temporary (short-term) memories we make are stored temporarily in the hippocampus of the brain until we go to bed. However, the hippocampus can only hold a certain amount of memories and information. So, when we sleep, these memories get transferred into more permanent storage.

Losing sleep piles pressure onto your memory-saving mechanism. It overloads your short-term memory and causes you to either be unable to retain memories or acquire new information. If this carries on for too long, you will also lose the chance to use deep sleep to consolidate and arrange your memories neatly.

- **Stress And Inflammation**

Sleep helps you stay within your physical and mental limits. Losing some hours of sleep once in a while may not necessarily count for much in the long run, but if you consistently get too little sleep, you run the risk of leaving your stress-coping mechanism permanently switched on. How? When you task your body beyond its limits (by not getting enough sleep), the body produces excess cortisol also known as the stress hormone to provide you with extra physiological abilities to cope with the stress. However, consistently-high levels of cortisol put more pressure on the blood vessels and increase blood pressure. Cortisol also induces inflammation within the tissues and vessels, and this can be the precursor to a stroke or other systemic failures. A 2013 study published in the *World Journal of Gastroenterology* noted that reduction in average sleep quality and length causes an upregulation of inflammation markers like Tumor Necrosis Factor and Interleukins I and 6. This directly links sleep deprivation with diseases such as Inflammatory Bowel Disease, Ulcerative colitis, and some forms of cancers.

- **Weight Gain**

People who sleep for a fewer number of hours are at a very high risk of gaining weight. A study led by Shahrad Tahredi and published in *Plos Medicine* found out that reduced sleep was directly proportional to an increase in Body Mass Index (the most reliable tool for charting body weight).

The mechanism by which this happens is not fully understood, but a 2011 study linked a disturbed balance of ghrelin and leptin hormones with reduced sleep. These hormones are responsible for generating feelings of hunger and satiety respectively. So, when they are disturbed, that means you will continue to eat without feeling full when you should. Shahrad Tahredi's team also corroborated this. They found out that in sleep-deprived people, ghrelin was significantly elevated and leptin was reduced. That means if you are sleep-deprived, you are likely to continue to eat beyond your usual limits. The extra calories you consume this way contribute in a big way to increase your overall weight.

Away from hormonal balance, there is a higher risk that you will eat more the longer you stay up. You need to provide metabolic fuel to keep yourself up for the extra hours you spend, and that means eating more. Late-night snacking, as a habit, is more common among people who sleep late at night. Since most of the food we eat at night is often processed foods, there is a chance that you will overload on the salts and sugar that are usually integral components of most processed foods. All these point to the fact that reduced sleep can lead you towards obesity. To cap it, as reported by a 2008 study published in *Sleep,* children and adults who get too little sleep have an 89% and 55% chance of becoming obese respectively. This practically means that inadequate sleep is a key cause of obesity.

Obese people are in even more delicate waters when it comes to sleep quality. Inadequate sleep can cause you to gain weight, and the extra weight you gain can make it harder for you to enjoy even the little sleep quality you get. This creates a vicious cycle of events that continue to lower the amount and quality of sleep you can get daily. Obese people are also more prone to a class of sleeping

29

disorders known as sleep apneas characterized by obstructions and swallowing while sleeping. Obese people find it harder to fall asleep and wake up more frequently during the night. Things are even worse if you gained a lot of weight in a short time. You may have further trouble adjusting to your new weight and that can further affect your sleeping posture. So, sleeping well is a baseline therapy for weight loss.

- **Diabetes**

When we consume sugar from our food (mainly in the form of carbohydrates), they get broken down into simple sugars (mainly glucose) and are absorbed into the bloodstream. Now, for the body to use glucose (our primary metabolic fuel), it needs to be taken up by cells from the bloodstream. This process is mediated by insulin, a hormone produced in the beta cells of the islets of Langerhan (in the pancreas). The absence of insulin makes it hard for our body to utilize the glucose present in the bloodstream. This leads to elevated levels of blood sugar as glucose remains in the bloodstream (this is also known as hyperglycemia). Now, diabetes is primarily characterized by hyperglycemia and the consequences of persistently high sugar levels. Diabetes can occur due to the body's immune system destroying the beta cells in the pancreas to stop insulin production. Another form of diabetes occurs when the cells cannot recognize insulin and the insulin produced is unable to help you utilize the glucose in the bloodstream. Diabetes, if left for too long, can cause severe eye problems, kidney dysfunction, fainting spells, a slowed ability for wounds to heal and even death in severe cases.

It's no news that reduced quality and quantity of sleep can increase the chances of developing diabetes, especially type 2 diabetes. However, how does a lack of sleep tie into diabetes? Well, we have already established that inadequate sleep causes weight gain, but did you know obesity is the most significant risk factor for diabetes? Yes, that is right. Women with a BMI above $35kg/m^2$ for instance, have 93 times as much chance of developing diabetes as women with a normal BMI. Apart from that, obesity causes fat deposition which can interfere with certain cellular organelles and result in insulin resistance. A 2010 experimental study further lends credence to this theory. The reports stated that a

31

week of sleep deprivation reduced mean insulin sensitivity among participants by as much as 24%. That's a significant figure in the scheme of things. Another study has also shown that glucose tolerance is negatively affected by sleep deprivation. These mean that better sleep will help you defeat the odds of coming down with diabetes mellitus.

- **Cardiovascular Disease**

Paul Walker, foremost sleep therapist has stated that "Adults above forty-five years old, who sleep for fewer than six hours are twice as likely to suffer a heart attack as those who sleep for more than six hours." His position is further buttressed by another study that showed that shorter sleeping duration could cause cardiovascular complications. Yet another review of 15 different studies showed that people who sleep for less than seven hours on average have a significantly-increased chance of suffering a heart attack or stroke.

- **Cancer**

When you sleep late and increase the amount of light you are exposed to before sleeping, you inadvertently reduce the production of melatonin. Now, melatonin is a hormone that not only regulates sleep; it also reduces the chances that you will develop cancer by suppressing the growth of tumors. If you delay your sleep constantly then, you run a greater risk of developing both benign and progressive tumors. Learning to shut down your body in accordance with its usual cycle may be the difference between great health and having to deal with full-blown cancer.

- **Sleep And The Immune System**

The immune system is our body's innate defense system that works to eliminate most infections and reduce your risks of coming down with an illness. Now, the strength and efficiency of the immune system differ from individual to individual and sleep is one of the factors that can determine just how strong and effective your immune system is.

A study published in *JAMA* revealed that sleep deprivation can increase the risks of septicemia, among other immune dysfunctions. This buttresses the point that not getting enough sleep can compromise the

33

immune system leaving you susceptible to all kinds of infections. In people with poor sleeping habits, a reduced humoral response has also been reported to vaccination. Aside from the length of sleep you get, when you sleep is also an important factor. The immune system relies on a network of cytokines, chemical messengers, that control cellular and humoral response to potential infections. Most of these cytokines exhibit a diurnal variation, peaking in the early hours of each day. If you are fond of going to bed very late, you run the risk of distorting this rhythm and compromising your health. A separate study in *FASEB* also showed that even partial sleep deprivation can lead to a significant reduction in the total number of available white blood cells, natural killer cells, and lymphokine-activated killer cells. This means that most of the cells involved in the immune response are significantly reduced by a lack of sleep.

Inadequate Sleep And Mental Health

Mental health refers to your ability to stay in control of your thoughts, emotions and beliefs as well as possible.

Emotionally-healthy people are able to compartmentalize their feelings and they realize that present emotions do not need to push them to act rashly. Getting adequate rest and sleep is one of the basic ways of maintaining good mental health. The effects of inadequate sleep are immediately noticeable on mental health and the level of emotional control you are able to exhibit. If you sleep poorly, it is likely you will wake up cranky and feeling unrefreshed. That alone can set a lot of loose reactions off within your mind, leading to unwanted complications and impaired judgment. Some notable effects of poor sleep help to potentiate the following mental health disorders.

- **Anxiety Disorders**

If you suffer from an anxiety disorder, then you should always strive to get enough sleep daily. Anxiety and panic disorders often have triggers that may be activated by how you are feeling. Feeling drowsy or fatigued even in the early mornings can leave you on edge, and it would require just a gentle push to get you into a panic attack. When you sleep well enough, you would be able to cope better with your emotions, by observing and

35

acknowledging emotions that come up rather than being in a reactive state. It may not work all the time but staying fresh and relaxed can help you reduce the frequency of anxiety attacks you get. You simply do not want to go about with a heavy head if you have a history of anxiety disorders.

- **Bursts Of Anger**

Yes, we all wake up cranky when we have not gotten enough sleep. Grogginess and the weariness that comes with not getting enough sleep can leave you with a shorter fuse than usual. You are likely to be more sensitive and irritable to any perceived slight and delay. That may manifest as regular outbursts of anger that you may even regret later. However, if you are sleeping poorly, these outbursts can become a semi-permanent fixture of your routine and affect your relationship with other people.

- **Depression**

Depression and its alleviation represent a significant portion of attempts to boost mental health worldwide. If you have ever been depressed, you will realize just how lonely one can get when his thoughts have him in jail. It's a terrible feeling to be lonely even in the middle of a crowd, and sleep has an impact on that too. In fact, that last phrase is an understatement. As reported in the *Journal of Clinical Psychology,* nine in ten patients suffering from depression present with complaints about their sleeping patterns. In an even more recent study, 33% of respondents suffering from insomnia reported depressive tendencies occasioned by their inability to fall asleep quickly enough.

The link between depression and poor sleep actually follows psychology logic. For most depressed people, nighttime offers the best chance for them to do their overthinking without being disturbed. Lying in bed is often the trigger for negative and self-deprecating thoughts to come flooding into their mind, and processing these thoughts puts them in a mood where it is hard to source for sleep. This leads to generalized insomnia and with time, if uncontrolled, the normal sleep cycle gets disturbed severely. Being unable to sleep well further entrenches a feeling of gloom and doom for depressed patients during the day as they have a go at their tasks in less than optimal mental conditions. Therefore, insomnia is often a recurrent feature in depression and should be a focus of intervention in any therapy for depression.

Good sleep is a tonic for good mental health. It allows you to turn in each night ready to unload your worries, doubts and fears. It is a chance for you to divest yourself of all the emotions that might have dogged you throughout the day.

Effect On Productivity

Sleeping well enables you to get up each morning, ready and alert to go complete your tasks and goals. When you sleep well, you will wake up with a spring in your step that can take you anywhere you want to be. You will get up in high spirits and beam smiles at everyone you meet along the way. That will also afford you your usual quota of energy, reducing the needs for a quick-fix or soft drinks. Waking up fresh will help you get to sleep later at night as scheduled. You do not want to carryover sleep debt to the next day, or it will just get compounded.

38

Sleeping late, on the other hand, has been implicated in a sharp reduction in performance. That shouldn't come as a surprise. Nobody performs well with a raging headache and drowsiness. That also explains why a lot of driving accidents occur early in the morning or late in the evening when people are most drowsy.

Poor sleep is a big problem that you should look to fix as soon as possible. It can lure you into unproductivity and actually get you used to the lowered performance levels.

Chapter 2: Get in Synch: Your Body's Internal Clock

Why do you get sleepy at night? How does your brain know when it's time for sleep? How does it know when it's time to get up in the morning?

The answers to these questions lie in a clever mechanism devised by the body to regulate its activities – the circadian rhythm. Many chemical and biological activities in the human body reach peaks and troughs under the guidance of the circadian rhythm. In sleep, the circadian rhythm represents the body's biological clock that allows our body to cycle between periods of wakefulness and sleep effectively.

Every day, our body runs a cycle that causes us to feel sleepy around the same time each day if it remains undistorted by external factors. The circadian rhythm works in a way that allows a dip in energy twice in a day – from around 2:00 am to 3:00 am and between 1:30 pm and 3:00 pm. These periods are marked by a general decrease in energy levels and alertness. Often, you may not notice the early morning drop since you are most likely asleep during that time, but the afternoon drop is definitely noticeable. It is responsible for that post-lunch lethargic feeling and for why most people opt for afternoon naps, without really understanding the cause for this recurring midday sleepiness.

The circadian rhythm aims to keep you in a defined cycle that allows you to get maximum rest while sleeping. In people who work night shifts, for instance, logic dictates that they try to get some shut-eye during the day to leave them refreshed for the night shift, but this hardly works in that way. Most shift workers have reported that they find it hard to sleep during the day to compensate for their lack of sleep at night. This is because their bedtime clashes significantly with their internal clock. Trying to sleep during the day goes against the natural inclination to stay awake, and working through the night infringes upon the natural circadian rhythm.

You may be wondering at this point why and how knowing about the circadian rhythm is of any importance to you.

Well, the circadian rhythm is the most important control mechanism that the body employs to control your sleeping pattern. Most people, however, unknowingly go against this internal clock. This results in a distorted sleep pattern that can drain one of his vitality and alertness in the short term.

The rhythm itself is controlled by the hypothalamus (in the brain), and most of its efficiency in establishing a sleeping pattern is related to light. How? The retina in the eye has special cells that conduct light and help us tell when it is nighttime. Once it is dark, they pass this information to an area of the hypothalamus known as the Suprachiasmatic Nucleus (SCN). This information tells the brain that it is time to sleep. In blind people, extrasensory measures are employed to get to the same conclusion that it is time to sleep.

The SCN communicates with the pineal gland (located between the brain hemispheres) to release melatonin, which is also known as the sleep hormone. The moment melatonin is released, the body gets ready to sleep. If you are not ready to sleep, it then becomes hard to stay awake. You may start to yawn, your eyelids may begin to feel heavy, and you generally feel inclined to hit your bed at that moment.

That is when you may say that you are sleepy and need a cup of coffee, or any other stimulant to stay awake. What these stimulants do is to try to rouse the brain from "sleeping mode" – this does not even work all the time. After some time, your body is just going to get used to the amount of caffeine you take and render it ineffective as a stimulant. To reinstitute its stimulatory effect, you may need to increase the amount of caffeine you consume at once leading to further biochemical imbalance. Even then, yes, you may succeed in delaying your sleep at this point, but each moment you spend awake after that requires you to use work against the body's natural inclination. At other times, even double the usual amount of caffeine not going to keep you awake, especially when you are suffering from sleep deprivation.

The circadian rhythm can get disturbed on a short-term basis, but it doesn't really change in the long-term. Napping in the afternoon, for instance, can cause you to feel more alert than usual at night and stay up longer than usual, but the moment you stop napping in the afternoon, your natural inclination to sleep at night gest restored promptly.

It is important to follow your circadian rhythm as closely as possible to ensure you get enough rest. Sleeping at odd times makes it very hard for you to enjoy the therapeutic effects of sleep. Think of the times you have stayed up at night, only to fall asleep in the early hours of the morning. Did you feel as sufficiently rested as you should have? Definitely not! That's why you need to construct your sleeping cycle with respect to your natural rhythm and try to keep your bedtime as consistent as possible.

Keeping a regular bedtime has a lot of physiological importance. A research study published in *Scientific Reports* concluded that an irregular sleep pattern actually increases the risks of developing metabolic diseases like obesity, hypertension, and heart diseases over the next decade. This implies that you must pay attention not just to the average length of your sleep but also how regular your bedtime is. The golden rule used to be "Sleep for an average of eight hours daily," but scientific evidence also suggests that we should actually have a set time to rest.

That throws up the question, "When is the ideal time to sleep?"

To answer this question, I will need to first explain the different stages of sleep we pass through.

The Sleep Cycle

A century ago, there was no explanation for the contrast in the quality of sleep different individuals enjoyed. The differences include how long it takes to fall asleep and why the same individual slept deeply at times and only lightly at other times. The invention of the electroencephalogram (EEG) in 1929 provided clear evidence that a sleep cycle is present in humans and other living things. The EEG (much like the ECG used to monitor heart activity) records brain wave activity to explain our sleep pattern. The findings provided proof of the existence of a sleep cycle.

Even without the EEG to show us how we go through different stages of sleep, the signs that we do abound. Physical signs such as eye movement, different levels of awareness, and muscular movement while sleeping lend further credence to the sleep cycle that we all follow.

There are four sequential stages of wakefulness, light sleep, and deep sleep regulated by the brain to bring about sufficient rest each night. This sequence forms a cycle between the two main types of sleep we have; the Rapid Eye Movement (REM) and the Non-Rapid Eye Movement (NREM) sleep. REM sleep as the name would suggest features rapid, uncoordinated movement of the eyeballs while we sleep, which is not found in NREM sleep. Typically, the first kind of sleep we go into is the NREM sleep followed by REM sleep. The NREM sleep features three stages that give way to REM sleep to complete a cycle that takes 90 minutes on average. Let us look closely at these stages.

Stage I (NREM1)

The moment you lie in bed and start to fall asleep, there is a general decrease in wakefulness and brain activity. The frequency of the brain waves decreases until you reach NREM1, which is characterized by alpha waves of 9-13 Hz. At this stage, you feel very relaxed and in a resting phase. You are definitely not awake, but you aren't really asleep either. It is easy to get startled and awaken in this stage by external interference. If someone wakes you up in this stage and tries to talk to you, it is likely you won't remember. This stage lasts for one to seven minutes and is often called the alpha stage because of the predominant alpha waves.

ⵜ Stage II (NREM2)

NREM2 is characterized by light sleep. Eye movements, muscle contraction, and general metabolism slows down even further. There is a more even tone of breathing, and you are fully asleep. Theta waves appear at this stage, and the frequency of the brain waves is further reduced. Towards the end of NREM2, larger brain waves (high amplitude, small frequency) begin to appear. The entire stage lasts 10 to 25 minutes.

Stage III (NREM3)

The high-amplitude waves first seen in NREM become larger and dominate completely at this stage. Also known as delta waves, they signal a very deep sleep from which it is hard to wake up from. The entire body is relaxed, and brain activity is quite low. NREM3 occupies the largest part of our sleep cycle and lasts between 20 and 45 minutes on average.

Stage IV (REM)

REM sleep is characterized by high brain activity, almost at the same level as when we are fully awake. Immediately after NREM3, brain activity begins to increase. In fact, there is a brief ascent into NREM2 before REM sleep takes over. It is in REM sleep that most dreams occur. You are likelier to remember your dreams if you get awaken during this stage. There is also a marked increase in muscle contraction. Yet, we stay temporarily paralyzed as a protective measure to prevent injuries that arise from sudden movement of body parts.

Putting It All Into Practical Use

Every night, we are expected to complete about four to five cycles with an average duration of 90 minutes shared unequally among the different stages. For instance, the first few cycles feature extended NREM3 stages and NREM1, NREM2 and REM sleep typically lengthen with each successive cycle. Coupled with your knowledge of circadian rhythm, it means you can create the perfect sleeping routine and know exactly how long you need to sleep for, daily. The key points to note are (i) to sleep early, in accordance with the circadian rhythm, and (ii) avoid waking up during the sleep cycle.

It is best to awaken nearer the end of the sleep cycle or at least towards the end of the REM cycle. For one, this allows you to get up at a time when brain activity is almost similar to what you get while awake. That will prevent the pounding, groggy feeling you get when awakened from a deep sleep.

In practical terms, you need to set your alarm to wake up after the last completed cycle. Since each cycle lasts about 90 minutes, you can time your alarm appropriately. For example, if you're going to bed at 10:30 p.m., and need to wake up at 6:30 a.m., set your alarm clock to 6 a.m. instead to account for the 90-minute sleep cycle intervals. Even though you lose 30 minutes of sleep, your body will feel more rested, having woken up after completing REM sleep.

You also need to factor in sleep latency. Sleep latency refers to how long it takes you to fall asleep or get to NREM1 on a normal day. You should add a latency period to your calculations to ensure you do not mess with the cycles. For instance, in the example above, if it takes you an average of ten minutes to get to sleep, you should consider sleeping at 10.20 pm instead to account for sleep latency. Not factoring in those 10 minutes will distort your calculations. Kindly note that taking a nap during the day affects sleep latency – of course, it is going to take a little longer to sleep at night if you have taken an afternoon nap.

There are many sleep cycle clock applications available for Smartphones – they help you calculate when you should get up each morning. Some of them can even be synchronized to the default alarm clock on your phone or serve as alarm clocks. You can also use https://sleepyti.me/ to calculate how much sleep you should be getting and the ideal time for you to get up without breaking an active sleep cycle.

Remember, the key goal is to sleep at a regular, predefined time daily and to sleep in multiples of 90 minutes. That can make all the difference in how alert you are in the mornings and how much rest you get from your sleep.

Chapter 3 : Finding Your Perfect Match: Tracker or Diary?

Getting a good night's sleep can be hard, as you know. Too much exposure to artificial light, distractions and noise are only some of the factors that can deprive you of good sleep. However, it doesn't matter whether you are a very busy parent or an overworked student. You can still use a good night's sleep.

Despite the need to stay awake and hang out with friends on social media or check your office mail before going to bed, the consequences of not getting good sleep are far-reaching. Poor sleep can increase your risk of developing undesirable conditions ranging from hypertension to diabetes, heart diseases, drowsiness, and a general drop in physical performance levels. That is exactly why you need to know how much sleep you are getting on average. Or do we?

Is It Beneficial To Track Sleep?

Tracking your sleep will provide you with data that lets you know how you are getting on in bed, but the data may actually just be mere estimates which do not represent the realities. Most trackers measure inactivity to represent sleep. They have sound and motion detection abilities, and the moment these cease, they assume you are asleep. That may not be necessarily true though – sleep latency has to be factored in too. Aside from the possibility of skewing sleep data, though, there is another pressing concern about tracking one's sleep.

Yes, tracking your sleep may provide you with a lot of data, but then, what do you intend to do with the data? A school of thought argues that tracking your sleep can be counterproductive as it may lead to anxiety in the face of sleep. Dr. Kelly Baron, a clinical psychologist from the University of Utah, questions the value of the data generated. According to him, "(most people) …are not sure what to do with the data or the data ends up making them more anxious."

Nevertheless, I believe realizing you have a problem is the first step in solving that problem. Although there may be slight errors in the data generated, tracking your sleep provides you with a clearer view of your sleep patterns. It is practically impossible for you to know this if you do not track your sleep. The question of what to do with the data is easily answered too. If the data you have generated says you are not sleeping well enough, then that raises awareness within you that you need to work towards sleeping better. Secondly, your tracking system can also help you to monitor whatever form of therapy or treatment you choose to reposition your sleep.

However, you must pay attention to ensure that gathering data about your sleeping habits does not become more important than actually sleeping. This is a more common problem than you may think. Some individuals with wearable sleep technology pay extra attention to them when they awaken briefly at night. Their interest in knowing for how long they have slept and if they are hitting the right spots can prove to be of disadvantage to their sleep. As with everything, moderation is key, and tracking your sleep should not become more important than sleeping itself.

Potentially, it is important to track your sleep, as a prelude to optimizing it. We tend to become more aware and deliberate when we track our performance. So, tracking your sleep can help you uncover whether you are getting sufficient sleep or have to improve your sleep routine. In order to ascertain which strategy works perfectly for you, it is imperative to device a modality to keep track of your sleep data. Such findings will provide further insight on which you can reflect upon and improve your sleep, both quantitatively and qualitatively.

Now, how can you track your sleep?

There are two major ways to track the amount and quality of sleep you are getting; (1) Sleep trackers and (2) Keeping a sleep diary.

Sleep Trackers

The increasing frequency of sleepless nights and stressful days in the life of the average individual has made sleep tracking increasingly popular and useful. Luckily, technology has caught up to provide us with different options to track our sleep with. In fact, sleep tracking technology is fast becoming an industry on its own. The rave these days is about measuring all body indicators possible. From heart rate to breathing rate and the distance we cover daily; some solutions can help us track our overall performance.

Although sleep trackers are available in various shapes and sizes, they all generate the same kind of data that can be organized into well-detailed charts showing sleep duration. People who are worried about their lack of sleep are more likely to purchase a sleep tracker now more than ever. These trackers (mostly wearable) can help you determine if you are getting the right amount and kind of sleep. They provide data based on the generalized measurement of your sleep against the average of others.

Appropriate use of trackers will add value and additional insight to help you sleep better. Some sleep trackers even contain soundscapes, or bedtime stories designed to help you fall asleep. Trackers can also provide useful tips and raises personal awareness levels for great sleep. More advanced versions also make claims of helping to determine just how restless or restful your sleep was by accounting for the periodicity and frequency with which you toss around the bed. Also, sleep trackers can help you analyze the quality of your sleep environment. They can factor in lighting and sound levels to determine if you are sleeping in optimal conditions.

Some sleep trackers also calculate how much time you spend on each stage of your sleep – most of these come with inbuilt alarms that try to wake you up at the end of your sleep cycles. As I have mentioned in the first chapter, it is important to wake up at the right time. However, I must mention that no tracker can actually monitor your sleep cycle with a hundred percent accuracy. This is because the different stages of sleeping are best monitored with brain activity, and an EEG is the best, most accurate way of doing that.

Sleep-related issues such as snoring can also be better managed using sleep trackers. With them, you can say farewell to the grogginess that comes with waking up because the smart alarms they come with, rouse you at the best time possible to keep you better rested and ready to go. That alone can be the difference between a productive day and an unproductive one.

You must note that sleep tracking devices are not a one-size-fits-all solution to all sleep problems, but they are a handy tool in your armory. They can even help a certified sleep therapist to devise better solutions customized for your needs. If you are the kind of person that relies on metrics to achieve your goals, then making use of a sleep tracking device is essential.

However, if you get stressed out easily when it comes to tracking your health indices, it may be better for you to adopt a sleep diary as an alternative means of tracking your sleep.

Using A Sleep Diary

A sleep diary is an alternative and simpler means of measuring your sleep pattern. For all that a sleep diary is, it is simply a personal record of your sleeping habits, and activities carried out before sleeping. You may be asked to keep a sleep diary by a medical professional, or you may decide to do so for personal benefits. Unlike sleep tracking devices, sleep diaries require you to put in practical, manual work to track your sleeping habits.

A sleep diary contains different types of data such as,

- Time of last significant activity before going to bed
- Time of consumption of last food before going to bed
- Amount and time of alcohol consumption during the day
- Duration and number of times you wake up at night
- Length of an afternoon nap
- Subjective evaluation of your feeling when you wake up in the morning

59

More data can be included in the sleep diary, depending on the individual as there is no stipulated or official format for a sleep diary. Making use of a sleep diary doesn't require any formal training or experience, either. An average individual can discover his/her sleep pattern with the sleep diary. However, it is imperative we let medical professionals such as doctors and psychologists observe our sleep diary as they have more experience. Sleep diaries can be used by people prone to insomnia, anxiety, sleep disorders, or those who do not fancy the idea of wearing a tech tracking device.

A sleep diary helps you monitor the effectiveness of your treatment if you have a sleep-related disorder. For instance, if you are suffering from sleep apnea, your physician can actually confirm his/her suspicion with the data provided in your sleep diary. The individual can also monitor his/her progress and response treatment by comparing the data of the pre-treatment and post-treatment period. Knowledge of your progress and positive response to treatment may further spur you to continue treatment, especially when you can readily see the results.

Although in using a sleep diary, you won't encounter the encumbrance of sleeping with a tech device, you must, however, note that writing about your sleep in a diary can be time-consuming and demanding. Furthermore, the accuracy of your data entry may be lacking in integrity as you may be in doubt over certain values and time. It is fairly common to forget to complete the entries when due and rely on your power of recall to complete them.

I get a lot of questions about which method is better for tracking one's sleep. It all depends on the individual – trackers are almost completely automated and can perform a wide range of roles and duties at once. They also require little to no input from you to compile the data they harvest into a meaningful form. However, they can be a source of anxiety and distraction while you sleep. Fiddling with them can take up some of the time you should use to sleep. Sleep diaries, on the other hand, require you to fill data from your observations manually. Sleep diaries hardly affect your sleep and offer you pretty little distractions. They are more helpful when you already have insomnia. This means each method has certain strong points and advantages over the other.

A Third Option?

So, who says you cannot combine both? Yes, I advise people to combine both unless one causes more harm than good to the individual in question. Yes, it is possible to use both methods at once – you can take a tracker along with you to bed and keep your sleep diary close to you as well. This will ensure you can tap the benefits of both methods.

Combining both methods will help you validate the data from both. That will remove some of the fears of inaccurate data. You will also be able to obtain data that encompasses the objective and subjective experience of sleep. While the sleep tracking device provides objective data, the sleep diary provides more subjective data.

Top Tracking Devices

In recent times, top tech companies like *Apple* and *Fitbit* have manufactured devices designed to monitor and help improve the sleeping habits of their owners. To this end, there is an extensive and wide variety of sleep tracking tech devices. There are enough to get one confused. Not all sleep trackers are even wearables these days; they come in different shapes and forms. To help you sort through a lot of the technical specifications better, I will list and describe some of the best sleeping trackers out there for you.

✦ *The Fitbit Versa 2*

Built on a 1.4-inch OLED bright screen, the Fitbit Versa 2 boasts of accuracy and reliability in measurements. New models are equipped with Alexa voice assistant, which makes it possible for you to set alarms, make searches, and give instructions to the tracking device with your voice. The Fitbit app further presents data of your sleep stages using a clearly detailed graph. More so, you could actually use the Fitbit Versa 2 to store about 300 songs. Personally, I have used one in the past and it did deliver on the promises. However, I am a bit worried that some of the extra features it carries may serve as potent distractions while one is in bed.

✦ *Beautyrest*

If you aren't comfortable wearing a tech device to sleep but yet want your sleep to be tracked then, Beautyrest is the perfect device for you. Beautyrest is a contactless tracking device that lies under your bed. With a measuring pad, a data processor, and a smartphone app, you can be assured that every toss and turn is being recorded. The device also tracks the heart and breathing rate. It is also equipped with daily lifestyle questions and suggestions on how they affect your sleep. Beautyrest is quite easy to use – you do not even need to be tech-savvy. With detailed and clearly illustrated graphs, it also saves you the stress of scratching your head and wondering what the data provided means.

Withings Sleep

This tracker has undergone a rather interesting evolution from the first time it appeared. Just like the Beautyrest, Withings Sleep is a contactless tracking device placed under your mattress. It subsequently transmits your sleep data to your smartphone. It is also very easy to set up both the app and the tracking device. What more? It *claims* to provide a detailed measurement of your sleep stages and reveals the total time spent in each stage and the percentage. If you also have sleep-related issues such as snoring, then Withings Sleep is a great option to consider, as it also records snoring and heart rate.

✦ *Beddit 3 Smart Sleep Monitor*

This is a dedicated sleep tracker that makes use of a thin strip placed under your bedsheet. It is used alongside a smartphone app that reveals the wide range of sleep information garnered by the tracker. Latest versions of this device record information such as snoring, bedroom temperature, and humidity. The Beddit Smart Sleep Monitor also tracks heart and respiration rates.

✦ *Oura Ring*

This tracking device is designed especially for those who do not fancy placing a tech gadget under their mattress or wearing it on their wrist. The Oura Ring provides you with data of your simple sleep score every day, your heartbeat rate, and the amount of movement your produce while sleeping. It is designed as a ring to be worn on the finger, and it can blend in easily without being a

65

distraction or intrusive. While many wearables are designed as activity trackers, the Oura Ring's main purpose is for sleep optimization, therefore its data is said to be more accurate than other competitors, which is also reflected in the price.

Tracking one's sleep is the first step in learning the right sleeping habits, identifying issues and fixing them. Minor issues can be addressed by focusing on your sleep routine & hygiene, but if your data suggests a deeper problem, then consulting a professional will be necessary in order to provide adequate treatment. On the other hand, you may discover that you are already on the right path and only need to stay consistent with your current bedtime routine. Tracking your sleep is also one of the easiest daily tasks you have ever had. If you cannot decide which method to choose between trackers and a sleep diary, you can actually combine the two to make one compensate for the shortcomings of the other.

Chapter 4: Lights On, Lights Off!

Light is perhaps the most important external factor when it comes to how well and how long you sleep. Light exposure has the potential to affect sleep both in the long-term and short-term. The relationship between light and good sleep is a curious one – it can be both a friend or foe, depending on how well you can optimize light. To get the best sleep possible, it is important to manage your exposure to light effectively.

To start with, let us look at why light is so important in sleep. Light can affect the quality of sleep you get both directly and indirectly. Directly, light can prevent you from falling asleep quickly. Leaving your lights on is more likely to cause distractions and give you new excuses for not going to bed immediately. Beyond that, light has always been a signal to stay alert and awake. As a race, we developed with clear demarcations that taught us that nighttime was for sleeping. The Ancient Man hunted and gathered fruits during the day, and once it was dark, he simply went to bed. Our bodies are not different from those of our ancestors, but the environment we now live in, has evolved much faster than the one our ancestors lived in. Nonetheless, it doesn't matter whether you think you are a night owl, our nights are made for sleeping. When you leave your lights on or stay in a well-lit place, you are conditioning yourself to find it harder to get to sleep.

I have discussed the role of the suprachiasmatic nucleus in the preceding chapter. It's the body's internal clock for regulating sleep via the secretion of melatonin. Unfortunately, light is its biggest inhibitor. It is the absence of light that causes the cells in the retina to send signals to the SCN to increase the production of melatonin and get the body ready to sleep. This is followed by dwindling metabolic rates and a reduction in body temperature. Therefore, the longer your interaction with light at night, the harder it is going to be for you to fall asleep. Research has shown, in fact, that light can

68

inhibit melatonin production by up to 85%. That is a marked decrease that has some potential significance to your sleeping pattern. Indirectly, exposure to light at night can also throw the circadian rhythm out of sync with your sleep cycle.

Is Light Totally Bad For Sleep?

With the amount of damage that light can purportedly do to your sleeping pattern, you would be forgiven for thinking light is definitely bad for sleep but that would be wrong. Instead, it is the time of the day at which you are exposed to light that determines if it will harm or boost your sleep potential.

In fact, the golden rule is to get as much light during the day as possible and get as little as possible at night. This follows the normal day/night routine, and more importantly, it dovetails nicely enough with the circadian rhythm. In fact, as supported by a study in 2014, light can help you calibrate your circadian rhythm better. The same study suggested that even blind people will get sleeping benefits from being exposed to sunlight during the day.

Getting enough sunlight during the day helps your hypothalamus differentiate out day and night properly, and prepare you efficiently for the night ahead. The more intense and the amount of light you get during the day, the clearer your circadian rhythm becomes defined. It also makes darkness function as a very effective signal to sleep.

Light also seems to increase brain activity and keep you alert. Making sure to dull things off at night, therefore, can help you get slower brain waves into action, to promote the amount of sleep you will get. It is also important to get natural light as opposed to artificial lights.

Illuminance, a measure of the intensity of the light given off by a light source (after considering distance and business) in lux (as a unit), gives us a great idea of how important natural light is during the day time. For instance, home lighting is at an average of 80 lux, and fluorescent light is around 320 lux. Consider these to the sun that has an average of 32,000 to 130,000 lux, and one begins to understand how important it is to get enough sunlight during the day. Sadly, this is not always possible or feasible due to work conditions. Most workspaces are illuminated artificially and that does not do enough for your sleeping pattern. Now that you know, maybe it is time to step out of that office once in a while to get a bit of sunlight. It is even better if you have a window; just try to look out of one as many times as possible daily.

Out With The Blue Lights!

If sunlight during the day is good for sleep, then the inverse is also true for artificial lights at night. As technology progressed, we learned to make light ourselves and use it for our needs. The problem is that the abundance of artificial lighting around us at night makes it harder to enjoy sleep of good quality. Among the different kinds of lighting we use, blue light is definitely the worst when it comes to interfering with sleep. Blue light is found in virtually all types of screens. It is especially common in smartphones, tablets, and personal computers. During the day, blue light is useful on these screens to calibrate sunlight exposure and make it possible to use the screens under intense sunlight. It has also been shown to improve attention span and lift your mood imperceptibly.

However, as night falls, it becomes a danger to good sleep. The fact that it is optimized for arresting our attention is its biggest drawback at night. Sadly, most people surround themselves with blue light in the moments leading to sleep while trying to read from phone screens or watch the television. Exposure to blue light drastically lowers the amount of melatonin produced in your brain, thereby keeping you up for longer than you want.

Practical Tips

As I have explained, there is a crucial need to optimize the amount of light you receive during the day and at night. The solution is for your exposure to light to reduce as your bedtime draws closer. Here are some practical tips to optimize light.

⚜ Get Your Daily Dose of Sunshine

Do not be caught cooped up in dimly-lit areas throughout the day. Get some sunlight into your system as frequently as possible. Sunlight is quite easily the best choice of light because it is readily available and brighter than any other source of light. A 2008 study by Nathaniel Mead lends weight to how beneficial sunlight exposure can be, especially in the morning. Based on systematic reviews, it is advised that everyone should get at least 30 minutes of sunlight in the morning. It wakes you up properly and helps calibrate your circadian rhythm. If you already have problems falling asleep, then 45 minutes should be your lower limit every morning.

On a gray or overcast day, when the sun is not even shining intensely, you can still get 10,000 lux of sunlight. This is many times more than what any commonplace appliance or lighting can give you. So, plan your day to include a lot of sunlight exposure. Walk to a nearby restaurant for lunch instead of getting it delivered, for instance. Spend some time reading on your porch instead of using your library. Just get some sunlight. You will be grateful you did!

♦ Consider Light Therapy

Light therapy can actually help you deal with some sleeping disorders. Special artificial lights that can generate up to 10,000 lux are available to help reset your circadian rhythm. Philip Sloane and his study group reported that light therapy is quite effective in the treatment of insomnia. From their findings, you only need to sit at a distance of sixteen to twenty-four inches beside a 2,500-lux light source for two hours or a 10,000-lux source for thirty minutes or place them in your living room to receive benefits similar to what sunlight provides. Light therapy can also help patients suffering from Seasonal Affective Disorder, a form of depression where symptoms are more prominent during winter and recede during summer. One explanation for this is that delayed daybreak in winter affects the circadian rhythm of such patients. As such, light therapy can help them recalibrate their circadian rhythm.

♦ Implement A Screen Curfew Two Hours Before Bedtime

I know. I know. It's hard not to surf the Web as you prepare to sleep. Or, maybe you like watching movies while waiting to drift off. I was guilty of trying to read eBooks too late in the night, but the fact is that you need to cut out as much blue light as you can. To do this, you may need to give up some of your habits then. That's a small price for the benefits that good sleep offers. Conservative researchers say one hour is a good enough limit for all blue screens before you sleep, but most scientists advocate that we are best served not looking at screens two hours before bedtime. So, you need to stop watching videos and reading eBooks while you wait for sleep to overcome you. You just might be delaying and denying sleep the chance to overcome you as quickly as you want. While waiting to drift off, consider reading the old-fashioned way. Yes, I am talking about holding a paperback book in your hand, a book that will require little alertness for you to follow, such as works of fiction as opposed to non-fiction.

Invest In Blue-Light Blocking Glasses

It is possible that you are unable to stay away from artificial light at night, perhaps because you work night shifts or require the usage of computers late at night. There are still measures to adopt in dealing with the efflux of blue light. Get yourself blue light blocking glasses and use them at night to reduce the light exposure your retinas get. At the very least, start using your glasses two hours before your bedtime. The basic blue light blocking glasses feature an orange tint that can deal with most of the blue light emitted from your devices. Wearing these will drastically reduce the amount of light-induced damage that is getting done to your sleep.

Turn Your Bedroom Into A Technology-Free Zone

I know that we all want our bedrooms to look awesome and offer maximum utility, but you need to stop turning your bedroom into a gadget store. The average bedroom these days boasts of semi-permanent gadgets like televisions and a wide array of lights, and more mobile tools like personal computers, tablets, and phones, that spew out a lot of blue light. The reason you are finding it hard to sleep may not be unconnected with the fact that you live in a blue zone that inhibits your sleep. It is called a "bed-room" for a reason – it is meant to be a place for sleeping and relaxation. So, leave your gadgets out of your bedroom and watch the difference in the quality of sleep you get. If you must bring in phones, keep them locked up in drawers where the blue light they emit will not escape from.

Devote Your Nights To Sleeping

Naturally, our nights are meant for us to sleep and unwind after working all day. If you can, try to keep your nights that way. Typical night owls feel their productivity is boosted at night due to a reduction in the number of distractions. That may have some merit, but it is a proven fact that brain activity is at its peak in bright, ambient light. That means we are mentally more alert during the day, and if you can deal with distractions, you will work better during the day.

Use Red Lights

Red light has a wavelength that makes it the best light to use at night. It affects circadian rhythm to a much lesser degree to all other types of light. Consider swapping the lights you have in your bedroom for red lights.

⚓ Turn Off All Lights 2 Hours Before Sleeping

Yes, turn them off! Forget the fact that you like sleeping with the lights on. They affect the amount of sleep you can get. The darker your environment is, the better the stimulation of the melatonin-producing mechanism. Darkness also reduces sleep latency significantly. So, turn off the lights at least two hours before you sleep so that you can fall asleep faster and enjoy your sleep.

In conclusion, light can be a great help or a potent hindrance to your sleep. Enjoy as much of it as you can during the day, and reduce the amount you get exposed to before going to sleep.

Chapter 5: Get Moving!

Everyone agrees that regular exercise provides us with a wide range of benefits. The whole world seems to be unanimous in the understanding that regular exercise allows us to enjoy better health and can even boost productivity. Yet, only a very small percentage of people get the required amount of daily exercise. Just like sleep, exercise suffers a lot once the average individual needs more time for other activities and tasks. Apart from time, many people are just not bothered about exercise, or a lack of it. Are you one of them? Well, if you are not getting regular exercise, let me give you one more prominent reason why you should be. Exercise helps you sleep better!

Charlene Gamaldo, the medical director of John Hopkins Center for Sleep, echoed the sentiments of other health professionals and sleep therapists when she said, "We have solid evidence that exercise does, in fact, help you fall asleep more quickly and improves sleep quality."

That has never been in doubt. There are no ironclad explanations for why exercise is linked to better sleep, but moderate to vigorous activities tend to get us exhausted, and sleep is usually the easiest way to recoup energy. Aside from that, exercise raises the core temperature of the body and in trying to cool off, that can evoke sleepiness.

Is Time of Exercise A Factor?

Everyone has their peculiarities and this often manifests in how our bodies may react differently to the same stimulus. With exercise, the timing could be important when it comes to its impact on sleep.

For instance, for some people, engaging in physical activities at night disrupts their sleep. This can be explained by the fact that exercise triggers the release of endorphins and other feel-good chemicals that lift your mood and cause you to stay alert. That's definitely inimical if it's close to your bedtime. For others, the timing of exercise seems to not have any effect at all on how quickly they can fall asleep. So, the best thing is to figure out how exercise affects you personally.

That exercise improves sleep is not in doubt at all. However, the timing could be everything as exercising late at night can extend your sleep latency and cause you problems getting to sleep quickly enough. A safe decision would be to stop all exercise about two hours before your regular bedtime. If you must exercise late at night, then be sure it doesn't affect your sleep. If it does, you need to cut it out of your night routine and find some time for it during the day.

How Much Exercise Do You Need For Better Sleep?

How much exercise should you look to include in your routine?

I have had clients who wanted to know how much exercise they should get daily and particular schedules for what sort of exercises to do to sleep better. My answer is always a variation of "…as much exercise as you can get without putting yourself in serious discomfort." There is no specific amount of exercise needed. Your target should be starting at your point of tolerance and working your way up gradually. I should stress that the effect of exercise on sleep is instantaneous. The people I have worked with have reported an immediate and noticeable increase in sleep quality on the days they exercise. Dr. Gamaldo has also validated this. She said, "It is generally not going to take months or years to see a benefit. And patients do not need to feel like they have to train for the Boston marathon to become a better sleeper."

The National Institute of Health recommends that you should get at least 150 minutes of moderate to vigorous exercise every week. You can spread that out over the week. Swimming, riding a bicycle, light jogging and a fast walk all qualify as moderate to vigorous exercise.

So, there you go. The way to get the best out of exercise is to factor what works for you, including the exercise type, time, and overall effect on your body and sleep.

Exercise For Chronic Insomnia

Chronic insomniacs get too little sleep, too frequently even when they invest time in trying to sleep. They either find it hard to go to sleep at all or wake up at night and find it hard to get back to sleep. Insomnia ranks as the most common sleep disorder among adults worldwide and is the subject of numerous researches and studies to help patients alleviate their symptoms. Results so far have shown a positive correlation between regular exercise and an improved sleeping ability in insomniacs. Moderate-intensity aerobic exercises such as walking, are considered the best options for improving your sleep.

Another way exercise works on insomnia is in its effects on your mental health. Insomnia is often a product or cause of mental health disorders such as excessive worry, stress, anxiety, and depression. Exercise improves your ability to combat these symptoms by lifting your mood. So, it can be a great tool for dousing depressive symptoms, clearing the mind, and relieving the body of stress. More studies are needed to understand the connection between exercise and insomnia fully.

In the meantime, more revelations (Kline, 2014 and Dolezal *et al.* (2017)) continue to show that increasing your fitness levels is one potent method of dealing with insomnia.

Creating Time For Exercise

Let's put aside sleep for a moment and talk about your exercise routine (or lack of one). It takes commitment and motivation to exercise regularly. I know this because I used to struggle with sticking to my exercise routine myself. Most people simply pick up exercise and dump it after a few days. January is particularly notable for how many New Year resolutions feature "getting fit" and "exercising". Yet, a poll by *Striva* has shown that most of these resolutions do not even last for up to two weeks.

Yet, the health benefits of exercise are too numerous to simply brush aside. Regular exercise improves cardiovascular health and boosts the immune system. That means you are less likely to fall ill when you exercise regularly. Exercise can even have a monumental effect on your social life. It can boost your confidence and perception of your body.

I think most people really understand and want the benefits of regular exercise, but very few people have the willpower to stick it out or create time for exercise in their daily schedule. Exercise is often one of the first casualties of a busy schedule. This does not have to be so.

Exercising does not mean you need to use the gym or spend an hour lifting weights. You can exercise in practically any space, and even ten minutes of exercise daily can give you most of the benefits you want. The best way to create time for working out is by choosing when it is most convenient for you. What works for you might not necessarily work for another person.

One way to make exercise stick for longer is to pick up a sport that interests you. It's easy to forget that you are getting exercise when you turn up at the neighborhood court in the evenings to play some basketball or kick a football around with friends. That way, you can wrap some social exposure with a hobby that gets you to exercise frequently. Also, you do not need much

85

equipment to exercise. Yoga, stretching, jogging, and skipping are all light exercises that you can achieve with the barest of sports equipment. Another useful tip is that exercise does not need to look like exercise. As an example, you can take little walks when you have been sitting for too long. You can use trackers that remind you to get up and walk around a bit every hour). Get off your chair periodically and walk around the office three times to get your body moving. Even that counts as exercise.

Three Simple Exercises To Do Before Bed

I will partially indulge your potential desire to know what exercises to incorporate into your night routine. Especially if you have not been getting any before, I'll recommend the following exercises for you. They are easy to start, require little facilities and equipment and can improve your sleep, starting from today.

Qi Gong

Qi Gong dates back to the ancient Chinese as a healing exercise. It focuses on breathing, meditation, body positioning, and gentle movement to put your body in recovery mode. The basis behind the exercise is that it aids the circulation of the "Qi," a vital energy force in the meridian system. By way of effect, the exercise also helps to regulate the body, mind, and breathing, thereby balancing the Qi. A study that took in 150 participants suffering from different mental health disorders, notably depression and chronic fatigue syndrome, has also revealed that Qi Gong can suppress insomnia, fatigue, stress, depression, and aid overall mental health. Best of all, it optimizes sleep latency and quality.

⚜ Yoga

Yoga has been a byword in healthy living for the last few years, and with good reason too. Yoga, as a physical exercise, plays on positioning and breathing to get you into relaxed positions that can improve body balance, tolerance, and reestablish a deep mind-body connection. A breakthrough 2013 study sampled 65 adults above 60 years old to compare the effect of yoga on the sleep patterns of those who practiced it. The total Pittsburgh sleep quality index score was much lower in people who did some form of Yoga compared to the control group.

This shows that regular yoga exercises can significantly improve sleep quality, even among the elderly.

There is also a wide range of Yoga poses to choose from. Balasana, Uttanasana, Ardha Uttanasana, Supta Baddha Konasana, Viparita Karani, Savasana, and Legs-on-a-Chair are only some of them. You may need an instructor or tutorial videos, in the beginning, to get them right, but there is surely a yoga pose out there for everyone looking to increase the quality of sleep they get at night. Youtube may be a good place so start your search for high-quality, and free 10-15 minutes yoga routines before bedtime, such as "Yoga with Adriene."

🔱 Tai Chi

I know – the first thing that comes to mind with Tai Chi are martial arts and fighting. Great sleep does not even appear at all, but that could be because most people do not know that Tai Chi can help them achieve that. Tai Chi isn't like most martial art styles– it features rhythmic breathing and mild meditation more than the usual kick-dodge-block-kick activities you would normally associate with martial arts. In fact, Chinese monks favor it a lot because it is easy to do – it is a particularly good choice for old-aged people, individuals that suffer from joint problems and/or limited flexibility.

A 2008 study published in the *Sleep* Journal by a team led by Dr. Michael Irwin, a professor of Psychiatry and Biobehavioral Sciences, corroborates the idea that Tai Chi can improve your sleeping pattern. A group of participants was asked to practice Tai Chi moves for 25 weeks, and the effects on their sleeping pattern were compared against another group that didn't practice Tai Chi. The result showed that participants in the Tai Chi group found it easier to sleep, slept deeper and woke up less frequently in the middle of the night.

Regular exercise must feature on your daily schedule if you really want to improve the quality of your sleep. It gets you going when you need more power and energy, and it helps you shut down faster and more effectively when you are ready to sleep. A win-win any day, all day long.

Chapter 6: Make it Sacred: Your Bedtime Ritual

Habits and routines make it easier for us to derive the benefits associated with certain actions. Drawing from that, creating a bedtime routine can make it easier for you to enjoy your sleep. The idea behind having a bedtime ritual is to alert your brain and body to prepare for sleep in advance. This enables you to have an external stimulus to create the perfect physiological conditions to fall asleep as soon as possible. A bedtime ritual should involve a sequence of at least five actions that will prepare you mentally for sleep. Your bedtime routine should also maximize your chances of falling asleep quickly.

I will now list nine core actions that you can and **should** incorporate into your bedtime ritual.

⬇ Set A Device Curfew For The Whole Family

This point builds on the tips I have covered about the impact of light on the quality of sleep you get. Since most gadgets emit light that makes it hard for one to fall asleep quickly, then, there is a need for you to set a curfew for operating electronic devices. That means no eBook readers, smartphones, or computers should be used once you have started preparing to go to bed. You should set a curfew that guarantees you at least a device-free hour before you sleep.

⬇ Take A Hot Bath 90 Minutes Before Your Bedtime

Many people suffer from high sleep latency that translates to an inability to fall asleep as quickly as they will like to. Well, hot baths can actually help you sleep better by reducing your average sleep latency figures. How does work biologically?

Without recourse to extra factors like illness, we run a temperature cycle in much the same way we run a sleep

91

cycle. Average body temperature often peaks around two in the afternoon and drops to its lowest figures while we sleep. Lowered body temperature while we sleep helps us to relax and rest better. So, finding a way to lower your body temperature in preparation for sleeping is a smart hack that you can achieve with hot baths taken an hour or two before sleeping.

When you take a hot bath, vasodilatation occurs. That means the blood vessels widen to bring more blood from within the warmer recess of your body to surface structures like the hand, feet, and face. The body seeks to establish homeostasis by rapidly conducting some of the temperature from the warmer blood to the atmosphere. Since a larger amount of *warm* blood is exposed to this effect, the body temperature can drop substantially by 3 to 4 degrees.

Shahab Haghayegh, the lead researcher in a study that looked at the findings of more than 5,000 reports of the connection between sleeping and a warm bath, concluded that "a warm bath led to more time spent in actual sleep rather than turning or tossing and trying to

92

fall asleep, compared to usual sleep without taking bath." The research team found out that warm baths of between 104- and 109-degrees Fahrenheit can promote sleep efficiently and help you fall asleep faster by about 36%. It is best to take this warm bath about ninety minutes before your usual bedtime to reap maximum benefits if you are looking for one way to reduce the amount of time you spend tossing around on the bed before you get carried away by sleep.

Consider Aromatherapy

The use of essential oils has been around for centuries, and ancient Chinese, Egyptian and Roman societies ascribed some of their most effective healing practices to these essential oils. Most essential oils play on our sense of smell to bring soothing and calming relief to the body in general. The nose as the sensory organ of smell is wired to directly drop its signals into an area of the brain that closely borders the emotion and memory center of the brain. That means scents can easily affect one's mood and play a part in our mental state. Most essential oils naturally stimulate the brain's emotional center and can bring you a more soothing rest.

Some of the more common essential oils include,

i. Lavender – Lavender is one of the most popular essential oils in the world today. Famed for its ability to reduce anxiety and induce a calm effect, it has been the subject of many scientific conferences and researches. Most of these researches are unanimous in agreement that lavender provides health effects in such areas as sleep optimization, depression management, and pain relief.

ii. Vanilla – Vanilla is another widely acceptable essential oil that produces a great scent. Beyond the pleasing scent, it has sedative properties that can help you fall asleep better.

iii. Jasmine – A 2003 research at the Wheeling Jesuit University led by Dr. Bryan Raudenbush has proven that jasmine can boost alertness during the day and help recalibrate the circadian rhythm for better sleep at night.

iv.   Rose and Geranium – Roses and geranium smell mightily nice and occupy a significant position in aromatherapy in terms of stress relief.

v.   Sandalwood – Sandalwood has been shown to increase the amount of NREM sleep and the management of anxiety symptoms. However, there's a caveat to its use. Sandalwood users have reported that it makes them active while relaxed. That may prove to be a problem for its use at night. If you have noticed that sandalwood leaves you alert and relaxed, then you should consider using it only during the day.

There are several ways you can use these oils to bring out the desired results. I will discuss three of the most effective ones here.

o   **Added To Your Bath**

You can add essential oils or a mix of different essential oils to your bath to maximize their effects. You can even soak yourself in a bathtub with drops of essential oils in the bath to get thoroughly immersed in their scents.

o **Diffuser**

You can use an automatic diffuser to get the scent of the essential oils into your room. You only need to put the essential oil and water in a predetermined ratio into the diffuser, then sit back and perceive the scent of your essential oil.

o **Direct Application**

If you like to go a more direct way, then you can also apply these essential oils to your clothes, skin, palm, or beddings directly. I do not advise direct skin application because of allergies but you can take things up a notch by applying essential oils directly to your bed, blankets, and other clothes.

Read Fiction at Night

Reading, at any time of the day, is a great mental exercise that can boost cognitive abilities and memory retention. It is one of the few ways of flexing our mental muscles and exercising the brain. Reading also boosts creativity and broadens one's knowledge base. Every moment spent reading is usually worthwhile and can be regarded as productive.

Beyond these well-known benefits of reading, though, did you know you can use reading as part of your ritual to boost sleep quality?

Yes, that's right. Reading a book before bed can relax you even further. It can take your mind off your worries and allow you a more even mental state to try to sleep in. I mostly advise my clients to pick fiction titles over works of nonfiction because fiction allows you more creative freedom. You can lazily allow your mind to wander, and you require pretty little mental attention to focus. Nonfiction titles may be a bit too serious and require more concentration than your body is really willing to lend. Reading such books may even make it harder for you to fall asleep because your brain is required to stay alert while you read.

How long you read for each night depends on you. I think maximum benefits can be reached when you do not make it a habit to continue reading until you fall asleep. Instead, decide beforehand the length of your daily reading habit. This will ensure that you do not get carried away by the books you are reading so much that you may go past your regular bedtime. It will also minimize the amount of light you get exposed to as you prepare for bed.

It is important to stress that hardbacks and hard copies are the preferred books of choice for a nighttime routine. This is because it is counterproductive to read from your phone, tablet, computer, or any other screen because of the blue light they produce. Good, old-fashioned books may be cumbersome or awkward to lug around, but they have the edge over electronic copies. Get one or two books to read, a few pages at a time, if you do not want to stack books all over your house. It is also important not to bring your books into bed. Why? Bringing books to bed will reduce your chances of falling asleep immediately and also create an association between your bed and a reading habit. This is counterproductive as you should ideally want your bed to be associated only with sleep and sex.

Try Meditation

It can be hard to switch off the mind when we get into bed. In those moments, while we wait to sleep off, a lot of thoughts pop up that seem to require immediate action, but the truth is that most of them don't. Paying attention to them can keep you awake for longer than you want. Mindful meditation offers you a chance to silence those thoughts as you await sleep. The 'goal' of mindfulness is to evoke a relaxation response, a mental phase where you are caught up only in the moment without thinking of the past or future. The hope is that the awareness of only your present circumstance will make you fall asleep faster.

As a therapeutic tool, very few techniques come close to the efficiency that mindfulness meditation can bring to the table. You can try to evoke the relaxation it offers by a variety of ways. I practice mantra meditation, but you can also apply visualization and even guided meditation to achieve a relaxed mind.

Here is a summary of the steps involved in the mantra meditation I practice.

o Pick a silent spot for your meditation and sit with your back straight, in the most comfortable position for you.

o Set a timer for 20 minutes (preferably one made for meditation, such as Insight Timer where you can pick softer ending bells at the end of the meditation to not be violently pulled out of your meditation).

o Exhale and inhale deeply a few times while paying close attention to all the movements involved in the process. Feel your diaphragms contract and relax as you breathe.

o Next, repeat a mantra you have chosen before starting. A mantra can be any word or phrase. In fact, it can be a meaningless phrase or word that cannot distract you. Repeat the mantra in your head as you continue to feel the breathing process.

o Inevitably, you will find your mind drifting off. Each time you notice this, kindly disengage from your new train of thought and return to the mantra. Do not feel bad if you drift off constantly or try to examine those thoughts.

- When the 20 minutes come to an end, stop repeating the mantra, and simply watch yourself take deep breaths for a couple of minutes. Do not skip this part, as going straight to a different activity after being in such deep meditative state can lead to discomfort and headaches.

You can also use visualization methods to achieve relaxation. Visualization involves the creative use of the mind to place yourself in a relaxed setting. For instance, you can picture yourself lying down alone at a beach, listening to the waves crash against the shore. Close your eyes, and try to soak yourself in the moment. Feel the silence and peace as if you were there already for a few minutes. You can choose a place you have been to or invent a new place completely in your head. The key is to choose a relaxed spot and then will yourself to be there. This mental safe and tranquil place can also be used as a go-to to seek refuge in, in moments of anxiety and stress.

You can choose any of the mindfulness or meditation exercises that appeal most to you. The most important thing is to be focused on trying to achieve the relaxation response.

◆ Play Music

Music is a universal language that is understood in every corner of the world. But perhaps, you have not heard of the health benefits that come with listening to certain kinds of music. Generally, music can help lift your mood, defeat stress, and create a renewed vigor and vitality. Slow music can also induce sleep and settle you quickly into your bedtime ritual. The key thing to consider is the rhythm of the music tracks selected. You may find it hard to sleep if you are listening to some soul-busting, adrenalin-inducing rap music. Instead, choose tracks that have rhythms around 60 beats per minute. As we sleep, the heart itself gradually settles into that range – listening to music around that rhythm can, therefore, help you reach deeper levels of sleep quicker. Notable songs that have such slow beats include the Marconi Union song, "Weightless," Joni Mitchell's "Blue Room Hotel," and

Miles Davis's "Blue in Green." There are many more out there that can help you sleep faster and deeper. I advise that you choose songs you are unfamiliar with or songs whose lyrics you do not know. That will ensure you don't end up singing along to the song for a large portion of your night.

✦ Give Journaling A Try

Just like reading, writing is a very effective form of therapy. It gives substance to the thoughts in your head and helps you clear your mind. It can be a great form of stress relief and help you rearrange your thoughts. Sleep is affected by your thoughts and mindset just as much as by any other thing. Journaling, much like meditation, helps you sort out those thoughts. One effective hack to apply while journaling is to show self-gratitude.

Write out the things you are grateful for – good health, a great family, a recent promotion at work, random acts of kindness – put everything you can remember down. Writing these down in your journal will flood you with positive emotions and endorphins that can boost your mood and uplift you. These will tune out any potential worries that you may otherwise take to bed with you and ensure you don't spend a lot of time tossing around with no sleep in sight. Aside from increasing the sleep quality you enjoy; journaling can also help you become productive. It can become a form of indicator for measuring your progress towards the goals you have set for yourself. You can pick that journal up in the mornings to create your to-do list for the day. Committing your worries, fears, and negative thoughts to paper halves their impact on your mood and emotions. Putting down the great things you have done or the things you are grateful for, cleanses your mind of worries and leaves you feeling awesome as you head to bed.

Put On The Right Night Clothes

When it comes to sleep, every single factor matters, from what you eat to when you turn off your television. On this note, it is important to ensure that you are dressed in as comfortable clothing as possible when you hit your bed.

When it comes to picking a nightgown or pajamas, the most important consideration is comfort. Nightwear

104

clothes come in different materials, with each offering certain advantages over the other. It's important to get conversant with the pros and cons of the most common materials before choosing what to slip into. Here are some of the more common materials;

o **Cotton**

Cotton is the most common clothing material. It is easy to touch, light, and breathable. It is also easily cleaned and if you are very interested in aesthetics, it lends itself well to pressing. Since it is also natural, it is highly comfortable with only one significant drawback in the area of insulation. Cotton is a very poor insulator and a poor choice in too cold and too hot temperatures. It doesn't keep the cold out when the weather is cold and that can give you chills that make sleeping uncomfortable.

o **Silk**

No material deals better with the elements than silk. Silk autoregulates your sleep experience in all kinds of weather. It keeps you warm when the weather is cold and is sufficiently breathable to allow you to lose body heat when the weather is hot. However, silk is rather expensive and relatively harder to clean. Because it is also slippery, it can slide around a lot while you sleep and generate static from free charges when the air is dry.

o **Wool**

Wool is sourced from animals, heavy and a great insulator that keeps out cold quite effectively. However, that also means that wool can leave you at the risk of getting over-heated – that can make you feel really uncomfortable even when the weather is cold.

o **Flannel**

Flannel is especially suitable for cold weather. It keeps you warm reasonably and allows air to circulate – that means you can stay all warm without feeling stifled.

o **Bamboo**

If you are trying to be eco-friendly, then this is the material for you. It is totally biodegradable and feels quite comfortable on the skin. It also absorbs moisture and limits perspiration to the barest minimum.

Aside from choosing the right material to wear to bed, you should also consider how tightly or loosely you want them to feel against your body. Your nightwear should be free enough to prevent chaffing or itchiness due to its tightness against your body. But it shouldn't be too loose, or you may find it sliding around you as you sleep, leading to uncomfortable sensations.

It is also important to consider your feet, hands, and head. If it is cold, you can pull a cap over your head or even consider gloves for your hands. If you don't, you may get uncomfortably cold, cold enough to disturb your sleep.

o **Sleeping Naked?**

There are distinct advantages to sleeping naked if the ambient temperature permits it. In warm weather, sleeping naked can help you stay cool. Of course, when you sleep naked too, you also eliminate the chances of uncomfortable clothing getting in the way. It is something you should really give a thought to – personally, I get deeper, more satisfactory sleep when I go *au naturel.*

⚜ Sex Before Bed

Yes, sex is good for better sleep. Anyone who has been in a sexually-active relationship probably already knows this. Sex causes a cascade of hormonal reactions that often leave you needing sleep at the end of the deed. It is a common joke that all men want to do after sex is sleep. However, it is not just men who often sleep better after sex; women do too. Aside from the effect of hormones, though, sex also promotes sleep indirectly by deleting most of the usual distractions that can disturb your sleeping routine.

The goal of a bedtime ritual is to get your prepared psychologically for sleep. For this reason, it is important that you make your routine an unwavering habit. You need to actually believe and be committed to the actions you have chosen for your bedtime routine and use them to the best of your advantage. By all means, feel free to switch one or two components but keep the core components intact, day after day.

Chapter 7: Setting the Mood:

Your Sleep Sanctuary

Now, let's address the physical space you sleep in. After the living room, people typically spend a lot on redesigning their bedrooms to taste. That's not bad at all when you consider the fact that, on average, we are expected to spend a third of our day sleeping in our bedrooms. For a place where we spend so much time, though, many people simply miss the main point. Your bedroom should be designed and structured with sleep as the central focus. I mean, it's all glossy and fancy to hang fairy lights left and right and install the biggest flat-screen television you can find, but all those things interfere with the primary reason our bedrooms serve – to sleep. Hence, you should be more interested in making your room a comfortable and peaceful place to sleep rather than a replica of a movie set or Blockbuster lookalike.

Making the decision to turn your bedroom into a sleeping room isn't always an easy one, but it's a cornerstone of this action plan. I remember how hard it was for me to come to terms with the fact that my large Sony speaker with its bright lights had to go out of the corner of my room. I convinced myself for the longest time that it actually served a practical purpose in helping me sleep, such as being able to play white noise or relaxing music before bed. I had to face the fact that this purpose could still be served from the living room instead.

Here are some points for you to note as you try to get around to making your bedroom conducive and healthy to sleep in.

⚓ Get Technology Out of Your Bedroom

I know I'm repeating myself but this is probably the most overlooked strategy there is. We all know that falling asleep beside our cellphones is bad, yet we still do it. If you only take away one thing from this book, then let it be this. Make it a tech-free zone. As I have echoed before, the mental associations your brain makes with your bedroom should be of only two things: sleep and sex. Notice how I didn't mention entertainment, therefore, that rules out television, tablets, and even books to some extent. It is fine to do those things before bed, especially reading if it's from a paperback book, but if possible, take it elsewhere. There is no excuse for leaving anything other than the most indispensable of appliances in your bedroom.

That brings up the question, "what appliance is indispensable in your bedroom?" To answer this question, simply get rid of every single thing that has nothing to do with sleep or personal safety. Yes, that includes your television, and even smartwatches (except sleep trackers). In particular, televisions make it harder for you to get to bed. In 2014, a team of researchers showed that televisions affected sleep even in school children. Another study in India in 2012, had earlier showed that people who stayed up in front of televisions reported shorter sleep duration.

Only appliances that are integral to good sleep should be left in a bedroom. This covers temperature-regulating appliances like air-conditioners and fans. You should also invest in models that make minimal noise and allow you to sleep in comfort. Electronic alarm clocks can also find a spot in your bedroom, obviously.

⚜ Do Not Bring Work Into Your Bedroom

Working in bed is bad for your sleeping routine. Working in bed completely alters the role of your bedroom. It subconsciously persuades your brain to believe that your bedroom isn't for sleeping alone. That can worsen insomnia if you already have problems falling asleep. Most often than not, work done in bed is of superficial nature. If you really have work to do, then stay up in another room to complete your necessary tasks before turning in for the night. Your brain should automatically start to scream "sleeping time" when you step into your bedroom. Do not leave it half-alert and unsure of whether you are about to sleep or work.

⚜ You Do Not Need That Nightcap

I will discuss alcohol and its effects on sleep in clearer detail in the next chapter, but I couldn't resist mentioning it here. Contrary to popular opinion, you do not need a nightcap a few minutes before sleeping. Alcohol is a potent drug that actively depresses the nervous system. That means it has the potential to mess with brain activity in the short and long-term. Yes, alcohol will sedate you initially, but it disrupts the duration of the stages in the sleep cycle later. It's hard to get a refreshing night rest under the influence of alcohol. There's a reason you wake up with a hangover the next morning after drinking heavily at night. Keep those bottles out of your bedroom.

⚜ Turn Your Room Into A Bat Cave

Bats are the gold medalists of sleep – they get an average of sixteen hours of shut-eye daily. One of the reasons they can do so is the details that go into the construction of their homes. Bats reside in cool, dark, and quiet caves that allow them to get good sleep with little chances of disruption. We can learn one or two things from them in that regard.

○ Get Blackout Curtains

Blackout curtains will, as the name suggests, block out light from the outside and keep your room dark as a bat cave. They are not always black, just in case black isn't one of your favorite colors for curtains – they come in different colors too and are cheap for the value they can offer your sleep.

o **Turn Down the Thermostat**

Temperature is a big consideration when it comes to sleep. Extreme temperatures affect sleep quality negatively. If the temperature is too warm, the chances that you will sweat and be uncomfortable increase significantly. Cold temperatures can also cause you to shiver or scrounge up in a position that doesn't allow you to sleep well. The ideal temperature you should try to aim for is between 60-70 °F. The body itself actively tries to get its temperature down as you aim to sleep. So, sleeping in a room at the ideal temperature will help you sleep faster and deeper.

o **Out With the Noise**

This is not rocket science – noise disturbs sleep significantly and can cause recurrent insomnia. Your bedroom should be as quiet as possible. That's why I advised earlier to get fans and air-conditioners with the lowest noise. Seek out all potential causes of noise in your surroundings and find a way to keep them silent at night or block out their noise. If you must keep your phones in the bedroom with you, remember to put it on silent to not be disturbed by notifications, be it by the noise or simply by the screen lighting up. If you live in an urban area where it is impossible to get quiet nights, invest in a white noise generator to minimize the effect of the sounds that get to you. Or quite simply, get some good, old-fashioned earplugs.

- **Pay Attention To The Air Quality In Your Bedroom**

As confirmed by research from the Annals American Thoracic Society, the quality of the air we inhale while asleep can determine how well we sleep. In particular, people who live in areas with a high incidence of air pollution were shown to receive sleep of lesser quality.

That means people who live in such areas are at a higher risk of health issues including decreased quality of sleep. Now, I know it may not be easy for you to ascertain just how good the air in your area is, but you can take steps to ensure the air in your bedroom is better. There is a need for your room to be well ventilated to allow efficient exchange of air at all times. Aside from that, certain plants can help you purify the air in your bedroom to a certain extent. Golden Pothos and Snake Plants, for instance, help to detoxify irritants such as formaldehyde, xylene, and benzene from the air around them. They also improve oxygen content and reduce the amount of carbon dioxide. Other beneficial plants include aloe vera, peace lily, elecampane, spider plant, and English Ivy. Except for aloe vera and elecampane, all these plants do not need direct sunlight.

⚜ Consider Changing Your Mattress

We spend a lot of time on our beds -literally, one-third of our lives. Unless you travel a lot or are have a lot of people you engage in other "bed-ly" activities, that means your bed is one of the constants of your sleep. It's surprising then how little attention we pay to the "health" and status of our beds. Most people only change their mattresses and bed for aesthetic reasons. The vast majority of people, however, use their beds past their best or are too unconcerned to know that their mattress is affecting their sleep.

Unless you have just moved houses or relocated, you will find it hard to remember the last time you changed your mattress. I am not chiding you – I am just making a point out of how much we ignore our mattresses. Now that I have your attention, what are some of the signs that the faithful servant that is your mattress is getting on in age?

- You sleep at the edge of your mattress to avoid a hollowed center
- Your mattress and bed creak and move with every move you make
- Your mattress has sagged considerably and lost the bouncy feeling it first gave you
- You wake up with severe back pains all the time
- Your sofa is as good a place to sleep in as your bed

- o You prefer to sleep elsewhere in the house
- o You sleep better in other people's bed or hotels
- o You can literally feel the springs or stuffing in your mattress when you press your back against it

A combination of these factors may very well point to the evidence that your bed is too weak to support your full form as effectively as it should. If you literally sleep "in your mattress" instead of "on the mattress," you are bound to lose a lot of the comfort a mattress is designed to give you. So, if you need a new mattress, you should seriously consider making the investment very soon. The primary considerations you should have in your mind should be quality and type of mattress material, your weight, and age.

Away from physical discomfort, do you know you are not the only occupant, rightfully or not, of your mattress? On average, there are ten million dust mites with you in bed any day. These little things feast on the dead skin cells you shed, and they "apologetically" leave their wastes on your bed since they cannot move very far. It is a pity that they and their waste products can generate allergic reactions that have been fingered as culprits in asthma, acne, dry skin, hair loss, and a dozen not-so-little disorders. You also sweat a minimum of a cup of water onto your bed most nights. That seeps right into your mattress and can cause mold and fungi to establish little colonies. I know all these are not your faults but it is a crime to allow the standards of your hygiene to slip when it comes to your bed manners. Wash your bedsheets as frequently as possible in warm water to rid yourself of unwanted visitors and their waste. You should also consider a waterproof mattress cover in the summer if you sweat a lot or live in temperate conditions.

What kind of mattress should you target?

There are various types of mattresses available for you to choose from. You might assume you have some ideas about them, but you will be shocked to realize how many choices you have to select from. To be honest, choosing the right mattress may become overwhelming if you do not have a firm idea of what you want before heading to a dealership. Now, what are your best shots?

o **Natural Fiber**

A lot of mattresses are manufactured with latex, organic wool, bamboo, coconut coir, and fiber. Coconut coir mattresses are often recommended for their quality. If you are particular about durability, consider organic cotton mattresses. Another option, Hemp mattresses, are often expensive and sophisticated. If you plan to host friends and you are interested in making your bed as attractive as possible, you should go for them. Bear in mind though that they are more focused on fashion than long-term service. You may have to change them in a few years.

o **Innerspring**

An Innerspring mattress is just what it is called—a mattress designed with inner springs and coils to help it firmly bounce when you jump into it. Continuous coils are the cheapest kinds of innerspring, but if you want something long-lasting and you are worried about cash, you should opt for Bonnet coils. If your priority is quality, however, you should consider Offset or Pocketed Coils. In particular, Pocketed coils are wired with springs at different points. This means if you bounce on one side of the bed, the other side doesn't rock. So, it is perfect if you have a partner, especially one who rolls about every time, even in bed. Regardless of the type, the best innerspring beds have a low coil gauge, about 15/12. Make inquiries about the coil gauge, and remember, the best innerspring don't sink.

o **Memory Foam**

Do you prefer to sink in your bed rather than bounce in it? Then, these types of beds are for you. The most interesting thing about Memory foams is that they give you such a comfy embrace that it would seem to be a hug. When you rise up from them, your shape is always clear-cut on the bed. Memory foams are also more resistant to allergens and dust mites and that's a plus you cannot overestimate. The only heartbreaking report about memory foams is that they trap heat as much as possible.

o **Waterbed**

Waterbeds are among the oldest types of beds around. They are exceptionally good for you if you are becoming bedsore for any reason. The major problem with a waterbed is how heavy they can be and how difficult it can be to set them up.

Silent, never complaining, and always loyal, maybe it is time to consider giving your mattress the fitting retirement it deserves. If you do not want to do it for your mattress, then do it for your sex life. Nothing beats a firm, proper mattress for sleep and sex.

⬆ Invest In A Good Pillow

We often overlook pillows, but they are an essential determinant of how well you are going to sleep. Many people focus only on the quality of their mattresses and neglect their pillows. Sadly, I have seen a lot of clients who suffer from totally preventable aches and pains that a good pillow might have prevented. While sleeping, you want to be supported and be as comfortable as much as possible, and your choice of pillow may decide how much comfort and support you get while you sleep.

It may surprise you to know that you are supposed to change pillows every 18 months. Yes! Experts believe that most pillows lose their ability to support your head and upper body after about a year and a half – that may even occur sooner than expected, depending on the quality of the pillow itself.

To test if your pillow is still in good condition, you can look for physical evidence that suggests it has done its time. In 18 months, the average pillow would have seen 8hours of action daily, and that is bound to leave telltale signs. Pillows also get a lot of dust, pollen, dead cells, and hair cells. That means if you do not change them as appropriate, you may be propping yourself up for allergic reactions.

One basic test to confirm if your pillow is still effective at what it should be doing is the fold test. Fold your pillow in half, then let go. Does it spring back instantly to its normal shape, or does it lay there folded? If your pillow has lost its ability to recoil back to shape when folded, that's an absolute sign that you are not getting the best of support from it, and you should get a new one immediately.

What kind of pillow should you get?

You will be making a mistake if you pick just any pillow without knowing its qualities. Some pillows are sleeping pillows, while others are special needs pillows for specific conditions such as sleep apnea, for example.

Factors To Consider In Selecting A Pillow

1. Filling

The first feature to consider is the filling of the pillow. What is it filled with? That can tell you a lot about how it is going to feel under your neck. In ancient times, people filled their pillow sacks with beans, stones, and the mildest of all, clothes. In modern times, you may choose between:

o **Down Feather**

Down Feather pillows are extra fluffy (maybe too soft than you'd like) but costly.

o **Memory Foam**

Remember the features of a sophisticated memory mattress? This pillow has those same features. They are cost-effective but can emit a nauseating odor (if not properly cared for) and traps heat.

o **Latex**

Latex pillows are synthetic pillows with almost the same features of memory foam pillows except that they are lighter, and offer greater comfort.

o **Gel**

Gel pillows are made from silicon materials. Their look, their touch, and their feel on the skin are entirely different from every other type of pillows mentioned perhaps because a gel cannot be classified as liquid or solid. This uniqueness alone can boost your comfort, offer premium pleasure.

2. Firmness

You definitely do not want a rock under your head nor banana peels. The firmness should be somewhere in between rock-hard and soft.

3. Size

The size of your pillow is as important as the other factors. You don't want a pillow that is easily one-quarter of your bed size or one so small it can barely support your head. Find a moderate-sized one. The standard sizes of pillows are;

    i.   14" by 20."

    ii.   20" by 26."

    iii.   20" by 30."

    iv.   20" by 36."

4. *Loft/height*

You need to consider the height of your pillow. You shouldn't choose a pillow so lofty you might get neckaches from sleeping on it. Remember, it just has to be moderate.

⚜ Choosing the Right Sleeping Position

Your sleeping position can determine how awesome your sleep would be. You naturally spend a lot of hours in bed, rolling and changing positions to get sound sleep. You must have noticed that you sleep better when in a certain position. Each time you hit this position, it doesn't matter if you are taking a nap or a long rest, your body just feels like you have hit the restart button, and you feel refreshed when you wake up. This is in contrast to other days when you wake up to creaking bones and a stiff back.

We agreed your mattress, and your pillow might have some say in the problem but your sleeping position plays an equally-important part too. You don't want to wake up every morning to excruciating pain in your neck when there is a stack of files waiting at work. There are so many daily tasks for you and starting the day with pain is the last thing you need. This is why you must pay extra attention to your sleeping position every time you crawl into bed.

Of course, there are lots of sleeping positions but you should not just jump into bed and curl into any form. Why? Not all positions are good or comfortable under the circumstances. For instance, a pregnant woman may ideally like to sleep chest down but logic suggests that her current state prevents that.

The most common sleeping positions are:

o **Flat On Your Back**

Lying flat on one's back is one of the most common and best sleeping positions people favor. It is a good way to rest your knees and thighs after a long day. Besides that, it relaxes the spine and core of your body. For extra comfort, you can even prop your knees up with a pillow underneath. However, if you have sleep apnea, you may need to prop another pillow under your head to enjoy maximum comfort. However, if you have back pains (due to sores, injuries, internal displacements etc), you will find it hard to go to sleep on your back.

O **Lateral Position**

Another common position is sleeping on one side of your body. It provides easy access to press phones, watch a TV, hold things, and discuss with a partner before you sleep. So, you must be cautious to ensure that this position does not encourage you to pick any of these habits that can affect your sleep negatively. Lying on your side also encourages light sleep allows you to react faster in an emergency much faster than lying flat on your back.

On the positive side, for people who snore, it is the ideal position because it makes it easier to breathe.

There is no conclusive evidence that sleeping on either the right or left side confers any advantage over sleeping on the other side. Lying on your side can also help you relieve back pains. You can even choose to put a pillow between your legs every time you go to bed to further alleviate back pain.

o   **Fetal Position**

The fetal position is a very popular sleeping position. It involves laying on one side (as in the lateral position) and curling your knees up to your stomach. Usually, your arms are around your knees. A lot of people revert to this position out of emotional needs, but it is also the best option if you snore heavily or are pregnant. Using the fetal position also has its own downsides though – waking up with cramps in the thighs, legs and abdomen is a common finding. Nevertheless, you can prevent stiffness or pains from your knees or lower abdomen by spacing your legs apart. Do not tighten the hold on your thighs, or curl intensely.

o   **Prone Position**

You can switch to the prone position by lying flat on your stomach. Your arms can be sprawled widely to both sides or kept by your sides. You can even hem your hands around your pillow, right above your head, or tucked under it. While this position is fairly common too and can help with snoring, it may not be the most efficient for you.

Firstly, if you have a big belly or have just eaten, sleeping on your stomach is an invitation to discomfort. In addition, you cannot keep your head, nose, and neck straight when you lay flat on your stomach; you would have to stick them to one side. That gives room for many niggles and stiffness upon waking up. You may also wake up more frequently than you would ideally want.

With sleeping position, comfort and balance are the most important considerations. Pick a position that suits your body shape and size and allows you to enjoy maximum relaxation. Your sleeping position should not bring you pain, cramps or stiffness. Experiment with different styles until you find the one that is most comfortable for you.

✦ No Animal Zone?

Should you keep pets in your bedroom or on your bed with you while you sleep? Well, a breakthrough study at the Mayo Clinic Phoenix found out that sleeping in the same bed with dogs does not affect your sleeping pattern. The study looked at the sleeping routine of 40 dog owners who allowed their pets to sleep in the same bed with them and found out that it did not interfere with the sleep quality they got.

This may differ from pet to pet, though. Dog are exemplary sleepers due to the fact they rarely turn and toss around while sleeping. In fact, if you turn and toss around a lot, you may find it hard to convince your dog to lie in the same bed with you. This may not be necessarily true for cats, for instance. Dogs may tolerate your movements better, but cats are naturally more alert and reactive than dogs.

Regardless of the pet you have, though, sudden turns from you may elicit sharp yelps or rapid movement from the pet that can awaken you. Other considerations should also come to play. This includes the temperament of the pet in question. Just like humans, animals possess individual traits even among the same breed. You should also factor in the familiarity between you and the pet. A new dog may not adjust to sleeping with you right away. You may need to bond for some time before both parties can come to a mutually-beneficial sleeping arrangement. I advise people with pets to try out what works best for them, in the knowledge that sleeping in the same bed with your pet does not mean you won't sleep well, but you must consider the peculiar temperament of your furry friend before making that decision.

Your bedroom should remain a sanctuary for you to turn to when you need sleep. You must preserve its sanctity by ensuring that it retains its primary purpose. Do not turn it into a home office, a spare library, a mini-cinema, a secondary dining-room, or anything else, except a bedroom. You will be happiest when it remains the sanctuary it is meant to be.

Chapter 8: Nutrition Habits: The Good, the Bad & the Ugly

No process in the body is not affected by what we put in our stomachs daily. Nutrition is a vital aspect and basis for all physiological reactions. The substances we consume are great determinants of how healthy we are. When it comes to sleep, our nutrition habits play an integral role too. When you eat, what you eat and what you shouldn't eat can all be crucial to the quantity and quality of sleep you get daily. Far too many people disturb their circadian rhythm out of sheer ignorance. For example, caffeine and alcohol, which have wide-reaching implications for sleep, are the two most widely used chemical agents in the world today. In this chapter, we will look at the effect of commonly-consumed substances and eating habits on sleep.

The Impact Of Caffeine On Sleep And Sleeping Patterns

What is caffeine? Caffeine is a natural brain-stimulating compound found in a diverse range of agricultural products, including coffee beans, cocoa beans, tea leaves, and kolanuts. Together, tea and coffee drinks represent 97% of the entire caffeine consumption of the world. Caffeine has also found its way into a wide variety of other processed foods such as chocolates, yogurts, soda drinks and energy drinks. People consume caffeine indirectly from these and many other sources of caffeine. However, the greatest reason why people consume caffeine is for its stimulatory properties on the brain. Or more precisely, its ability to keep one awake and alert for longer. The effects of caffeine consumption start to show in about ten to fifteen minutes after you have taken it. This makes it an obvious, quick-energy burst solution for most people.

Caffeine raises the body's metabolic rate which translates to an increased heart and breathing rate. Normally, we do not need caffeine in our diet, but it is not particularly dangerous either, especially when taken in moderate quantities. The FDA estimates "moderate" to be three 8-ounce servings that contain a total of 250mg of caffeine daily. However, the average American gets over 300mg daily. Especially among overworked individuals, coffee is a go-to option for delaying sleep and enhancing performance in short bursts. That is where the problem lies. In high doses, the stimulatory effect of caffeine can get so accentuated that muscle tremors, anxiety, panic attacks, dizziness, nausea and severe migraines may appear.

Of course, the most notable effect of caffeine is on sleep. As an adenosine receptor antagonist that blocks the release of adenosine, which is another important chemical messenger that promotes sleep, caffeine products are widely consumed to delay sleep. That comes with a lot of potential short- and long-term effects on sleep and energy levels.

Caffeine consumption at any time of the day can distort the normal circadian rhythm. If you consume coffee a lot, you must have experienced those swift and alarming drops of energy about five to six hours after its consumption. They are known as caffeine crashes, and they coincide with the time it takes for the body to clear half of the initial amount of caffeine you have consumed from your system. These crashes and the ability of caffeine to disrupt the circadian rhythm make it important for you to watch out for caffeine in your diet if you are having sleep problems. Caffeine addiction is a real threat, and withdrawal can present classic withdrawal symptoms such as mood shifts.

Tips For Limiting Impact Of Caffeine On Sleep

o **Adopt A Caffeine Curfew**

This is the most practical advice you can get when it comes to caffeine and sleep. Ban yourself from consuming all caffeine-containing drinks at least six to seven hours prior to bedtime. That way, the large portion of the effects of your morning coffee will have worn off by the time you are ready to sleep. Consuming caffeine, even late in the afternoon, can still have a sustained impact on your sleep, but by removing caffeine from your diet at least six hours before you are expected to sleep, you can expect to get better, but not optimal, sleep.

o Consume Caffeine In Moderate Quantities

If you must drink coffee or tea, then consider taking them in moderate quantities. Well, that is if you are not accustomed to a typical British or Swedish culture. I am only joking. The truth is that taking caffeine in large quantities has many negative health implications, including on your sleep.

o Are You Addicted To Coffee?

Most people can get weaned off their addiction to coffee on their own, but if you are finding it hard to do that, then you should consider seeking formal therapy for caffeine addiction. This may involve things such as Cognitive Behavioral Therapy or Neuro-linguistic Programming. It may even be as simple as reducing your workload so that you can function better without your morning coffee.

If you have any kind of sleeping disorder, then you should not even think of touching a single grain of coffee. It can greatly worsen things and reduce the quantity of sleep you get. Other than that, coffee consumed in moderate quantities, at least six hours before bedtime can be tolerated. The best thing, though is to stay off caffeine entirely at night if you are trying to enjoy better sleep. Or at the very least, go for decaffeinated coffee.

Dealing With Alcohol

Alcohol follows caffeine as the second most-widely consumed chemical agent worldwide. In contrast to caffeine, alcohol is a CNS depressant. At first glance, that would seem to mean that alcohol should help your quest to sleep off quickly enough, and that's true in a way. In fact, about 20% of Americans take alcohol to shorten sleep latency. The problem, though, is in the quality of sleep you get and the imbalance that moderate to heavy consumption can cause.

Technically, alcohol may make you fall asleep faster, but biologically, we can say alcohol makes you pass out (not sleep) quicker. Alcohol affects the usual array of hormones that regulate sleep. Notably, it boosts adenosine production. Adenosine promotes sleep; so, that is the reason why alcohol makes you feel drowsy and sleepy. However, alcohol is rapidly metabolized, and in as little as one to two hours, there is a significant crash in the levels of these hormones leading your body to feel more awake than it should.

Therefore, alcohol can cause you to wake up more frequently than usual, especially in the latter stages of the night. Alcohol is also a diuretic, and it causes the body to excrete more urine. Since adenosine levels are also reduced beyond normal in the later stages of the night, the bladder's ability to hold urine is also markedly reduced. That means more bathroom visits for you that can interrupt your sleep. As a muscle relaxant, alcohol can also cause the muscles around the neck and throat to function less optimally leading to airway obstructions, apnea and snoring.

Perhaps the greatest negative effect alcohol has on us is the shortening of the REM stage of the sleep cycle. At moderate doses, alcohol seems to have a limited impact on REM sleep but at higher doses, respondents have shown significant disruption. Even at low doses, though, there is a delayed onset of REM sleep. That means alcohol can deprive you of the restorative benefits of sleep. It may also explain why you wake up feeling tired, and all beat up after drinking heavily the night before.

In conclusion, alcohol at night messes with the circadian rhythm and promotes sleepiness during the day. It also causes you to sleep early but robs you of good quality sleep. So, it is in your best interest to stay away from alcohol at night. It does too little for the harm it can cause to you in the long run.

If you must drink, then, I would advise that you do so long about 4 hours before you plan to sleep? Why? The body metabolizes alcohol fairly fast. For instance, it takes one hour for the average-sized individual to metabolize a standard drink, which translates to 5 ounces of wine or 12 ounces of 5% ABV beer. Depending on the dose, 4 hours is a safe bet for your body to have gotten rid of the alcohol you have taken before sleep.

Are Sleeping Pills Safe?

Advil, Tylenol, Oxazepam, and the new "Z" class of drugs are popular sleeping pills used by a lot of people to get good rest, but do sleeping pills really work? Or, more importantly, are they safe?

Here's the gospel truth about most sleeping pills as corroborated by several research studies. The effects and efficiency of sleeping pills are exaggerated. They can reduce the sleep latency period, but using them only guarantees that you will sleep for just a bit longer than normal. In fact, a lot of the improvements that people have reported after using pills are due to a placebo effect. That means they felt or slept better because they believed in the power of the pill they took to provide that. So, they go to bed in the belief that the pills are about to make them sleep, and they do sleep.

However, these drugs have significant side effects that shouldn't be brushed aside. They can cause daytime

141

drowsiness, confusion, lost memories, and increase the risk of accidents associated with sleepiness. These effects are further exaggerated in older adults – their memories may be affected to a larger extent.

You are also required to continue using them for as long as you think you need them. That means you lose all the benefits they bring the moment you stop using them. So, if your insomnia prompts you to buy sedatives, remember that the moment you stop taking them, insomnia will return in full force. This throws up the potential for addiction. Benzodiazepines, the oldest type of drugs used as a sedative, are particularly addictive. You may find yourself helpless to stop consuming the medication even when you no longer need it.

Your body also grows tolerance steadily against the dose of medication you take. So, you may require successively increasing doses of the same medication to derive the same benefits. Now, this is where things can get out of hand. If you use them every night, they lose their effectiveness as brain receptors get used to their presence. With time, they literally stop working, and as

142

one researcher described them," they become as useful as a sugar pill.

The best way to use sleeping pills is infrequently. They have more potency that way and produce minimal side effects. They can help with jetlag and help you reset your internal clock. We will discuss more about reducing jetlag in the next chapter but in the meantime, here are a few rules to follow when it comes to sleeping pills.

- o Limit yourself to one dose per day. Do not take a booster pill because you are finding it hard to sleep in the middle of the night. It will have very little effect.

- o Do not combine sleeping pills with any other depressant or drug in general. Sleeping pills undergo a lot of drug interaction with other drugs that can cause unnecessary problems. In this regard, alcohol seems to be the biggest culprit. As a fellow depressant, alcohol potentiates the sedative effects of sleeping pills beyond safe limits. As reported by Ilomaki *et al.* (2013), this can result in accidents and an increased chance of an overdose.

o Do not take sleeping pills to sleep for a short time. Do not use sleeping pills when you just want to catch a few winks or sleep for only one or two hours. They are typically produced to knock you out for upwards of six hours.

o Avoid work that requires fine hand-to-eye coordination. Stay away from heavy machinery too, and do not attempt to drive until you are completely awake.

o Do not take sleeping pills if you have any sleeping disorder. Sleeping pills can further worsen the disorder by tampering with the biochemistry involved in hormonal regulation of sleep.

Melatonin And Sleep

A healthier alternative to sleeping pills is melatonin supplement pills. You already know the role that melatonin performs in ensuring that we get great sleep. Taking melatonin as a supplement can help stimulate your body to get ready for sleep. That is the difference between melatonin supplements and sleeping pills – it does not attempt to seize control of the entire sleep process; it just ensures that your brain gets the message that it is time for bed. Melatonin is also a powerful antioxidant that can deal with some of the oxidative stress within the body, raise growth hormone, and help to alleviate the symptoms of peptic ulcers.

By directly signaling the brain, melatonin supplements can help alleviate the effects of insomnia-promoting factors such as excessive exposure to blue light and stress. Analyzing the findings of 19 different studies also shows that melatonin supplementation can improve sleep latency by an impressive seven minutes on average.

Melatonin is also very safe, and non-addictive even in people who use it frequently. It does not distort the sleep cycle either. Nevertheless, I will advise that you start with lower doses of the supplement. You can try about 1mg of melatonin half an hour before sleeping to start with. If that does not yield productive results, increase the dose to 3 to 5 mg.

So, if you must take something to help you sleep, think of melatonin supplements. They are safe, easily available, and have minimal side effects. They promote a natural reaction in the body and do not distort the body's balance.

Cigarettes And Sleep

Smoking, in whatever form, is positively correlated with poor sleeping habits. A ResearchGate entry that studied 3,516 adults further established what many other reports have suggested in the past. No one is entirely sure why smoking seems to affect sleep, but it has been conclusively proven that smokers find it harder to sleep and wake up. So, they have extended sleep latency and need to sleep for longer to wake up refreshed. That aside, smoking comes with so many more health risks. If you are looking for better sleep, you may need to find a solution to your smoking problem. If you cannot let go of those cigarettes yet, then, at the very least, consider not smoking at least four hours before your bedtime.

Timing Food And Bedtime

Does everyone seem to have agreed that it is a taboo to eat right before going to bed? Well, that appears very logical from almost all points of view. Eating close to your bedtime means that you will be carrying a lot of undigested food and a distended stomach to bed. That can cause discomfort and make you feel heavier than usual. Apart from making it harder for you to sleep off, you may also find it harder to sleep deeper. Judging from this, it is certainly better if you eat about two hours before you sleep. This is supported by actual research that charted the impact of nighttime eating. That will give your body enough time to process and digest the food.

Spicy Foods

Spicy foods contain capsaicin and can actually raise your body temperature beyond the optimal range for good sleep. For this reason, it is better to eat them earlier in the day and drink enough water after eating a spicy meal. If you suffer from acid reflux or peptic ulcers, it is even more important for you to step away from spicy foods close to your bedtime. You do not want to trigger an ulcer attack or heartburn just as you go to sleep.

Does Eating Late Make You Gain Weight?

It is impossible to talk about eating late at night and not mention the myth that it causes weight gain. Let me burst that bubble for you – eating late at night does not necessarily make you gain weight. This is quite rightly one of the most contentious debates in the health world and it all depends on who you are listening to, but there has been no conclusive proof that eating late at night makes you grow fatter.

When it comes to weight gain, the difference between caloric intake and output is more important than when you eat. Indirectly though, eating late at night may cause you to wake up with a full belly and skip breakfast, leading to a higher chance that you will binge or indulge in junk foods high in caloric value later in the day.

You Cannot Go Wrong With Water, Can You?

Water is even easier to explain. There's absolutely no recorded evidence that drinking any amount of water can disrupt your sleep cycle. The only thing to consider is that drinking a lot of water close to your bedtime may cause you to wake up to urinate more times during the night.

To end this chapter, let me reiterate that what you put in your body is a very important part of your sleeping habits. Drugs and substances that can interfere with sleeping should not be taken close to bedtime or removed from your diet entirely. If it interferes with the quality of sleep you get, then it needs to go. So, consider stopping your regular glass of wine after dinner and stay off sleeping pills as much possible. Your sleep will be better for it.

Chapter 9 : Goodbye Jetlag!

Jetlag, also called desynchronosis or flight fatigue, is a temporary sleep disorder that usually results from quickly traveling across multiple time zones. Anyone that has traveled between different time zones knows how unpleasant jetlag can be. No matter how used you are to flying such distances, you will invariably end up feeling drowsy and lethargic for the first few days of arrival while your body catches up to the local time. What causes it?

When we move between different time zones, it's easy to adjust your watch, but the body's internal watch is less easily adjusted. For instance, if you land in Paris after flying from Miami (Paris is six hours ahead of Miami), all the eternal stimuli are telling you it's time to sleep, but your circadian rhythm is still effectively at 6 pm Miami time. That would mean you are trying to go to bed when your SCN is still telling your circadian rhythm it is not yet night. This imbalance will give you a metabolic jolt that can destabilize you for a few days until your internal clock is corrected. The word itself is coined from "jet" and "lag" – "jet" to represent the fact that air travel is the most practical way to move within multiple time zones rapidly and "lag" to represent the delay in the circadian rhythm.

Aside from fatigue, though, jetlag is also a potential cause of reduced performance and effectiveness – it can leave you in less-than-peak conditions, cause your negotiation skills to be off, and leave you unable to match performance expectations.

For frequent fliers, the symptoms of jetlag are all too familiar. Fatigue, insomnia, dehydration, and headache after journeying across time zones is mostly jetlag. Other symptoms can include diarrhea, waking up too early, constipation and grogginess, grumpiness, dyspepsia, confusion and malaise. Sometimes, temporary insomnia can be one of the symptoms, and these usually last for the first few days of arrival in the new time zone.

151

Why Is Jetlag More Severe When Travelling East?

Yes, it's not just your imagination. It is scientifically proven that you feel the effects of jetlag harder when you travel east than when you travel west. The 'why' is simple yet complex. In the body's internal sleep-wake clock, local bedtime comes earlier when you travel east and later when you travel west. For instance, Paris is six hours ahead of Miami. That is, 5 pm in Miami is equal to 11 pm in Paris. So, when your body is accustomed to the light-darkness cycle in Miami, and you suddenly arrive in Paris, it's like asking your body to sleep by 5 pm.

Meanwhile, when you travel westwards, you are asking your body to push harder and sleep later than usual. It's easier to sleep later than you're used to, compared to sleeping much earlier. That's why you tend to feel alert at night and then feel like sleeping all day. It is almost equivalent to staying up all night and then sleeping during the next day. Sleeping later and then waking up with the locals, or a little after them, is easier and results in lesser lag. When the lights are bright and the locals are still

152

bubbling, it gives you a feeling that the night is still young, and you can stay up some more.

Most people have a circadian cycle that is a bit longer than 24hours. This avails us more time to push forward. Conversely, it makes it even more difficult to track the clock backward, hence the banging headache you had to work with on your last journey eastwards. One other reason that makes it feel even worse is that the body has a lot of internal clocks that somehow find it easier to be pushed higher than lower. Even when environmental factors like daylight and activity levels manage to keep you awake when your body feels you should be sleeping, other clocks might beg to disagree. Several enzymes within the body that perform diverse functions, including digestion, may take a longer time to adapt to the new schedule. The lagging internal clocks then lose synchronization with those ahead, and that results in the sluggishness and feeling of exhaustion you get after making such journeys.

The good news is, you don't need to drag through the first few days of arrival at your destination. It could mar your purpose of making that journey. So, in this chapter, I've compiled some smart and effective tips that can make switching time zones a much easier task.

⬇ Modify Your Sleep Schedule

Adjust your bedtime before you embark on the journey. If you're traveling to a city that's three hours behind your usual location, you can adjust your sleep schedule and sleep an hour earlier each day for the last three days before your departure. If your normal bedtime is 11 pm for instance, then you should sleep at 10 pm, 9 pm, and 8 pm in the last three days preceding your trip. This technique has been scientifically proven to help in resetting one's biological clock as it kind of gives you a softer landing. Sometimes going to bed by 8 pm may seem too early, but taking the step to adjust will make your stay much better. When heading westwards, reverse the pattern by adjusting your sleep time by one hour. You may have to sleep later than you're used to, to beat the most significant symptoms of jetlag.

⬇ The Two-Day Rule

If you are on a short trip that won't last for more than two days, there is no point in trying to change your sleeping pattern. Why? By the time you adjust to the local time, it's time to repeat the entire process. Just buckle in for a rough few days as best as you can.

✦ Use Light Exposure

Light is one of the major regulators of your body's circadian rhythm, and a little tweak can help you adapt faster. If your circadian rhythm is saying you are at night upon arrival, get out and get some sunlight to remind yourself that it is actually daytime. That will help you recalibrate your circadian rhythm faster.

✦ Pay Attention to What and When You Eat

Eat meals at the appropriate local time, even if you aren't hungry. There will be the urge to eat by the time you've been used to but you must resist it vehemently. Eating high protein meals during the day when you hope to stay awake can be of great help.

✦ Optimize Sleep

The first few nights of your arrival should be optimized for sleeping. Limit things such as surfing the net and televisions that will keep you up unnecessarily. You don't want to move into a new time zone with a backlog of negative sleeping habits.

Exercise

Even little walks can help you stay alert and active throughout the day. It's true you may feel jaded from traveling but the benefits of exercising cannot be overlooked. Improved sleep quality and a much better social interaction are some add-ons that you stand to gain further from exercising.

All these tips can help you get acquainted with the new time zone faster but should only be applied if you are staying for more than two days.

Moderate Use Of Melatonin

Yes, sometimes, we just cannot afford to rest or relax upon arrival in a new time zone. That means we need a very quick readjustment, and many people turn to sleeping pills. You can do better though with melatonin supplements. We have discussed melatonin in the last chapter but then, I have to remind you of just how relatively efficient and safe it is.

As you know, melatonin is the hormone of sleep. It peaks about two hours before sleep and dwindles as daytime arrives. Melatonin can help reset your internal biological clock if taken as prescribed. If you are traveling east, and crossing many time zones, then, taking melatonin doses as high as 5milligram just before your trip is beneficial. It will help you simulate the conditions necessary for sleeping and help you mimic the effects of darkness on your sleeping pattern.

How To Get Some Shut-Eye On Buses, Trains & Airplanes

Simply because you are in transit on an airplane, bus or train doesn't mean you cannot get good sleep. Turbulence and constant motion may make it hard to sleep, but what if you feel the urge to doze off? The conditions may be less than ideal but nothing says you cannot enjoy decent sleep while in transit.

⚜ Find A Good Spot

First things first, it is very important that you find a good spot to fall asleep. You can try to find the most silent spots with fewer passengers – to avoid being disturbed by fellow passengers and their movements. If at all possible, I recommend choosing a window seat. You will be able to lean against the body of your vehicle and not have to stand up each time someone wants to exit or enter your row.

⚜ Reduce The Noise

While you sleep, your brain continues to register and process sounds on a basic level. Noise can, therefore, jostle your slumber, causing you to wake, move and shift between stages of sleep. An easy and quick solution to this problem is to get a pair of earplugs or sound-blocking headphones to reduce any background noise to a reasonable extent to ease your sleep.

⚜ Comfort Is Key

Ensure you wear loose clothes, and if possible, take off your shoes. If it isn't convenient for you to take off your shoes, loosen the shoelace. When traveling for long distances, it is advisable to wear cotton or loose materials that absorb less heat. By all means, avoid synthetic polyester as it would absorb more heat. If the air around you is likely to be too cool for you, be sure to dress appropriately.

⚜ Watch Your Sleeping Position

Your posture can also affect your sleep, especially the way you place neck – it is very important that you support your neck properly. You can try and lean on the window to avoid any unnatural bends to your spine. A neck pillow will be of good use here. Or you can try a jumper which can be rolled into a U shape and placed around your neck.

⚜ Block Out The Light

We all love to gaze outside to take in scenic views during our trips, but any daylight flooding through the windows will hinder your beauty sleep. Light is easier to block out on planes where windows have optional blinds.

However, it is somewhat trickier on a train or a bus. It is simpler just to cover your own eyes – an eye mask or even a pair of glasses will do the trick.

Trips and journeys, especially over long distances, are a part of everyday life. They take us outside our comfort zones and have the potential to disrupt the circadian rhythm. However, if you take the right precautions, you can not only minimize the effects of jet lag, you can also enjoy sleep of a similar quality to what you are used to.

Chapter 10: Now What?

Despite your best efforts, there are always those nights when sleep will elude you, or you find it very hard to go back to bed if awoken. This chapter contains practical tips for getting out of such frustrating situations.

Tips For When You Cannot Fall Asleep

Nobody is immune to this – I suffer from it too once in a while. It is possible to have prepared as best as you can for bed, yet, find sleep elusive. When most people have laid in their bed for about ten minutes without falling asleep, they get worked up and worried about what is going on. That, on its own, is a threat to sleep. Instead, when you find yourself unable to fall asleep, the ultimate goal should be mental relaxation – you may achieve this in two ways. One, you can employ any of the numerous breathing techniques to achieve relaxation or as I have found out, try to resolve the thoughts in your mind. I have come to realize that when I have a lot of worries or thoughts on my mind, my sleep latency period becomes extended. I know it's the same for everybody as the vast majority of my clients have reported the same findings. So, basically, what you need to do is try to calm your mind down and stop it from going to overdrive. The following tips should ideally help you do that.

⚜ Relax Your Mind

Try to shut off the little voices in your head. Do not allow fear and worry to hold your sleep to ransom. If there any pressing issues on your mind such as an important presentation at work the next day or a big decision you need to make, try to shift them out if they cannot be resolved. Keeping them on your mind is unlikely to solve them anyway. Now that you are in bed, your only concern should be sleeping. Try to get that into your mind. You can use guided sleep meditation, and nature sounds to help take the focus off from the internal chatter.

✦ Take A Shower

If you haven't yet done so, take a hot bath or shower. Sometimes, your inability to sleep is related to the ambient temperature. You can cover your body if the weather is too cold or turn the thermostat down to the optimal temperature for sleeping. A shower can also help you get to that temperature quicker. Plus, it gives you a chance to forget what's keeping you awake temporarily.

✦ Employ Visualization

This is one trick I have been using since forever, even before I discovered the importance of sleep. I simply allow my mind the creative freedom to wander and construct different scenes for me. I could be in Africa dancing to a soft, native melody one minute and listening to my favorite tune sung by an orchestra. I never stay in one scene for long, and I allow my mind to wander through positive images passively. I often find myself drifting off to sleep without even knowing it. It is important to ensure that you are not going through memories as that can quickly turn into an active process that requires mental concentration.

⚜ Address The Core Issue That Is Keeping You Awake

Why are you finding it hard to sleep? Most of the time, you will be able to find the answer to this. It could even be background noise, bright lights, or hunger. Try to fix what is keeping you awake if that is possible.

⚜ Get Up

If the tips above fail, then it is time to get out of your bed. Why? Trying to force yourself to sleep in such a situation may throw you into anxiety and worry. So, you need to leave your bed briefly to do something else. You can use that opportunity to do some basic chores such as folding clothes, or simply packing your lunch for the next day. Then, come back to bed after a few minutes and try to sleep again. The chances are that you will fall asleep straight away.

Tips To Fall Back Asleep In The Middle Of The Night

The average individual gets startled into waking up about four times each night – but we do not even remember most of these incidences by the next morning. A noise, a sharp change in temperature, or a pressing urge can get you up. Usually, once you have looked around and are satisfied that there is no immediate danger, you get back to sleep immediately. Sometimes though, this is not possible. What can you do in such situations?

⚜ Get Out Of Bed Briefly

Do not lie there counting the panels in your roof. Leave your bed and bedroom briefly into another part of your house. Think of that as restoring your sleep factory to its default setting. Find some little thing to do as you wait for your body to readjust. I usually read – one or two pages at most and then go back to bed.

⚜ Stay Away From Your Smartphone!

I know how tempting it can be to reach out and watch a video or two on your phone, but don't! That can ruin the rest of your night and make it impossible for you to go back to sleep at all. This is another good reason to keep your phone in a separate room – it is far too easy to simply grab it during those moments of tossing and turning. That applies to all devices around you, by the way. Shun them and focus on getting some shuteye.

↓ Don't Stare At The Clock

Whatever you do, do not stare at that wall clock and watch as it moves or count the seconds along with it. In fact, get your clock away from you or turn over until you can no longer see it. Counting the seconds will give you a sense of frustration and helplessness that can worsen your prospects of getting back to sleep.

In conclusion, whenever you are finding it hard to sleep, check within your mind to see if you have any worries or issues preventing you from going to bed. If you do, try to tune them out for the moment if there is no possibility of addressing it at that moment in time. If your mind is at rest, consider your physical surroundings and remove any potential disturbance. Turn off the lights and try to eliminate sources of noise. Then, close your eyes and allow visualization to take you on a journey to find sleep.

166

Conclusion

Sleep is one of the most important biological processes we need to function at optimal levels – it allows the body to recharge and regain some of its vitality. It is a chance to wipe the slate clean every night. It is a must that you enjoy as much sleep as you deserve. You cannot cheat human nature. You cannot negotiate or bargain time meant for sleep away. You should not use it for anything else.

Sleeping well, for long enough, can provide an instant performance boost. Knowing how and when to sleep and wake up can help you dredge productivity you did not even know you had. Good sleep will lift your moods and provide you with the emotional resilience needed to deal with tough situations we are all faced with. Best of all, good sleeping habits allow you to function like the real you – and not the groggy, unfocused, uncoordinated, angry version you have been lugging around.

Many factors threaten the quality of sleep you can get. Some are due to ignorance; others are due to our bad habits. Whatever the case, anything that affects your sleep has to go. The onus is on you to create optimal conditions for sleeping.

The first step is to assess your current sleeping pattern. How many hours do you sleep for, on average? When do you go to bed? Do you even have a specific bedtime? To do this, you can get a sleep tracking device and keep a diary. These will help you generate accurate data about what you need to improve upon.

Beyond tracking your sleep comes the heavy-lifting – repositioning yourself to enjoy maximum quality of sleep. To do this, you need to watch three things at all times – maximum comfort, a defined routine, and habits that promote good sleep.

Drawing from that, the message of this book can be summarized in three sentences.

1. Sleep in a comfortable bedroom with physical conditions optimized for sleep – think bat cave.

2. Develop a proper nighttime routine that ties in nicely with your circadian rhythm.

3. Build a catalog of positive habits that can enhance your sleep and remove all habits that have the potential to disrupt your circadian rhythm.

You must make your bedroom comfortable for sleeping. This starts with your bed and pillows – learn to choose the best materials that offer comfort to support your sleeping form. Learn a lesson from bats too – keep your bedroom as dark, silent, and cool as possible to enhance your sleep. Light exposure, especially blue light from screens, can make it hard for you to fall asleep. It can rewire the hormonal control of sleep and distort the circadian rhythm. No one sleeps well in noisy environments either and extreme cold or heat can make good sleep an unachievable target for you.

Make provisions to ensure that temperature changes are not too rapid or prepare against them in advance. Pay special attention to your choice of nightwear – the key target is for your sleepwear to be as comfortable as possible and hold up against the weather conditions. Air pollution can also provide long-term problems to your sleeping routine. So, avoid it as much as possible. If you live in an area where the air quality is particularly not good, consider using vents and windows to get fresh air in and out of your bedroom. You can also spare some effort to raise air-cleansing plants such as aloe vera, peace lily, and golden pothos. They remove some common air pollutants and toxicants and help fix more oxygen in their immediate surroundings. This can make a huge difference in the long run. Physical comfort is a golden rule you cannot mess with when it comes to sleep.

You also need to build a bedtime ritual that climaxes with you dropping into bed at a predetermined, regular time every day. Your bedtime ritual should ideally lead your mind to sleep. By starting with a bath, for instance, you are gently coaxing your body temperature into the ideal range for good sleep. Add essential oils and you are getting all the help available to make you sleep soundly in short order. Slow music, meditation, reading and even sex all gradually lead you towards satisfactory sleep. A device curfew limits the amount of blue-light you get and helps prepare the melatonin-secreting mechanism for optimal functioning.

Make your bedtime ritual a habit every day and you will find it easier to sleep deeper. The moment you start the first task on your ritual, your body initiates the sequence for shutting down. That means your body gets advance notice that you are about to sleep and can adjust accordingly. By mentally preparing your mind in advance, it is going to be mightily easier to fall asleep. So, do not just jump into bed the moment you decide to sleep. Instead, build towards a satisfactory close to the day's activities. Allow your system a chance to shut down gradually instead of trying to yank out the power cord and force it into sleep immediately.

Your habits have an integral role to play in the quality of sleep you enjoy – even seemingly unrelated habits such as how much water you drink and the kind of music you listen to can affect your sleep. Consider stopping the consumption of caffeine and alcohol if you have problems sleeping. If you cannot stop consuming them, then consume them in low quantities several hours before you sleep. The same thing applies to smoking and using sleeping pills. In our technology-laden world today, our devices often walk into bed with us. We take work into our bedroom and make it hard to sleep. These are habits you have to stop. Your bedroom has only two uses, sex and sleep. If you have something else to do apart from that, then you shouldn't be in your bedroom. Any other task can wait or be done elsewhere.

The take-home message from this book is that *"The bedroom is meant for sleeping, your physical comfort is key to a great night-rest and your routine and habits determine just how well you are going to sleep."*

Spread the word and allow this message to be the guiding principle for any decision you reach about your night rest.

Getting good sleep is a priority for everyone. For many people, though, good sleep is sadly elusive. They find it very hard to sleep for long enough to enjoy the restorative effects sleep is supposed to bring. Ignorance of the fact that they can do more to sleep better is a key factor. Luckily for you, ignorance is no longer in the equation. With this detailed guide, nothing can stop you from enjoying regular sleep, if you want it. You no longer have to toss around for eternity waiting for sleep. There is no longer anything stopping you from enjoying a deep, peaceful slumber every night. I have handed you the master key to great sleep. It remains to be seen how badly you want to unlock the door to more fulfillment, vitality, productivity, good health and vigor. You can literally reach out now and close your hands around "good sleep."

Are you ready to do that? Well, on your marks, get ready...sleep!!!

Resources

Ali, T. (2013). Sleep, immunity and inflammation in gastrointestinal disorders. *World Journal of Gastroenterology*, *19*(48), 9231.

Bankar, M., Chaudhari, S., & Chaudhari, K. (2013). Impact of long-term Yoga practice on sleep quality and quality of life in the elderly. *Journal of Ayurveda and Integrative Medicine*, *4*(1), 28.

Bonmati-Carrion, M., Arguelles-Prieto, R., Martinez-Madrid, M., Reiter, R., Hardeland, R., Rol, M., & Madrid, J. (2014). Protecting the Melatonin Rhythm through Circadian Healthy Light Exposure. *International Journal of Molecular Sciences*, *15*(12), 23448–23500.

Buxton, O. M., Pavlova, M., Reid, E. W., Wang, W., Simonson, D. C., & Adler, G. K. (2010). Sleep Restriction for 1 Week Reduces Insulin Sensitivity in Healthy Men. *Diabetes*, *59*(9), 2126–2133.

Cappuccio, F. P., Cooper, D., D'Elia, L., Strazzullo, P., & Miller, M. A. (2011). Sleep duration predicts cardiovascular outcomes: a systematic review and meta-analysis of prospective studies. *European Heart Journal, 32*(12), 1484–1492.

Cappuccio, F. P., D'Elia, L., Strazzullo, P., & Miller, M. A. (2009). Quantity and Quality of Sleep and Incidence of Type 2 Diabetes: A systematic review and meta-analysis. *Diabetes Care, 33*(2), 414–420.

Cespedes, E. M., Gillman, M. W., Kleinman, K., Rifas-Shiman, S. L., Redline, S., & Taveras, E. M. (2014). Television Viewing, Bedroom Television, and Sleep Duration from Infancy to Mid-Childhood. *Pediatrics, 133*(5), e1163–e1171.

Chan, J. S. M., Ho, R. T. H., Chung, K., Wang, C., Yao, T., Ng, S., & Chan, C. L. W. (2014). Qigong Exercise Alleviates Fatigue, Anxiety, and Depressive Symptoms, Improves Sleep Quality, and Shortens Sleep Latency in Persons with Chronic Fatigue Syndrome-Like Illness. *Evidence-Based Complementary and Alternative Medicine, 2014*, 1–10.

Cohen, D. A., Wang, W., Wyatt, J. K., Kronauer, R. E., Dijk, D.-J., Czeisler, C. A., & Klerman, E. B. (2010).

Uncovering Residual Effects of Chronic Sleep Loss on Human Performance. *Science Translational Medicine*, *2*(14), 14ra3.

Dolezal, B. A., Neufeld, E. V., Boland, D. M., Martin, J. L., & Cooper, C. B. (2017). Interrelationship between Sleep and Exercise: A Systematic Review. *Advances in Preventive Medicine*, *2017*, 1–14.

Ebrahim, I. O., Shapiro, C. M., Williams, A. J., & Fenwick, P. B. (2013). Alcohol and Sleep I: Effects on Normal Sleep. *Alcoholism: Clinical and Experimental Research*, *37*(4), 539` – 549.

Ellenbogen J.M. (2005). Cognitive benefits of sleep and their loss due to sleep deprivation. *Neurology*; 64(7):E25-7.

Francesco, P.C., Frances, M. T., Ngianga-Bakwin, K., Andrew, C., Ed, P., Saverio, S. and Michelle, A. M. (2008). Meta-Analysis of Short Sleep Duration and Obesity in Children and Adults. *Sleep*; 31(5): 619–626.

Gallant, A. R., Lundgren, J., & Drapeau, V. (2012). The night-eating syndrome and obesity. *Obesity Reviews*, *13*(6), 528–536.

Gooley, J. J., Chamberlain, K., Smith, K. A., Khalsa, S. B. S., Rajaratnam, S. M. W., Van Reen, E., Lockley, S. W. (2011). Exposure to Room Light before Bedtime Suppresses Melatonin Onset and Shortens Melatonin Duration in Humans. *The Journal of Clinical Endocrinology & Metabolism*, *96*(3), E463–E472.

Gottlieb, D. J., Punjabi, N. M., Newman, A. B., Resnick, H. E., Redline, S., Baldwin, C. M., & Nieto, F. J. (2005). Association of Sleep Time With Diabetes Mellitus and Impaired Glucose Tolerance. *Archives of Internal Medicine*, *165*(8), 863.

Guo, X., Zheng, L., Wang, J., Zhang, X., Zhang, X., Li, J., & Sun, Y. (2013). Epidemiological evidence for the link between sleep duration and high blood pressure: A systematic review and meta-analysis. *Sleep Medicine*, *14*(4), 324–332.

Haghayegh, S., Khoshnevis, S., Smolensky, M. H., Diller, K. R., & Castriotta, R. J. (2019). Before-bedtime passive body heating by warm shower or bath to improve sleep: A systematic review and meta-analysis. *Sleep Medicine Reviews*, *46*, 124–135.

Hayley, A. C., Williams, L. J., Venugopal, K., Kennedy, G. A., Berk, M., & Pasco, J. A. (2014). The relationships between insomnia, sleep apnoea and depression: Findings from the American National Health and Nutrition Examination Survey, 2005–2008. *Australian & New Zealand Journal of Psychiatry*, *49*(2), 156–170.

Ilomäki, J., Paljärvi, T., Korhonen, M. J., Enlund, H., Alderman, C. P., Kauhanen, J. and Bell, J. S. (2013). Prevalence of concomitant use of alcohol and sedative-hypnotic drugs in middle and older aged persons: A systematic review. Annals of Pharmacotherapy, 47(2), 257–268

Irwin M. D., Olmstead, R. and Motivala, S.J. (2008). Improving Sleep Quality in Older Adults with Moderate Sleep Complaints: A Randomized Controlled Trial of Tai Chi Chih. *Sleep*.

Irwin, M., McClintick, J., Costlow, C., Fortner, M., White, J., & Gillin, J. C. (1996). Partial night sleep deprivation reduces natural killer and celhdar immune responses in humans. *The FASEB Journal, 10*(5), 643–653.

Kinsey A.W. and Ormsbee, M. J. (2015). The health impact of nighttime eating: old and new perspectives. *Nutrients*;7(4):2648-62.

Kline, C. E. (2014). The Bidirectional Relationship Between Exercise and Sleep. *American Journal of Lifestyle Medicine, 8*(6), 375–379.

Li J, Cacchione PZ, Hodgson N. (2017). Afternoon Napping and Cognition in Chinese Older Adults: Findings from the China Health and Retirement Longitudinal Study Baseline Assessment.*J Am Geriatr Soc.*;65(2):373-380

Lunsford-Avery, J. R., Engelhard, M. M., Navar, A. M., & Kollins, S. H. (2018). Validation of the Sleep Regularity Index in Older Adults and Associations with Cardiometabolic Risk. *Scientific Reports, 8*(1).

Mead, M. N. (2008). Benefits of Sunlight: A Bright Spot for Human Health. *Environmental Health Perspectives, 116*(4).

Nag, C., and Pradhan, R. (2012). Impact of television on sleep habits. *Biological Rhythm Research:* 43. 423-430.

Patel, S. I., Miller, B. W., Kosiorek, H. E., Parish, J. M., Lyng, P. J., & Krahn, L. E. (2017). The Effect of Dogs on Human Sleep in the Home Sleep Environment. *Mayo Clinic Proceedings, 92*(9), 1368–1372.

Payne, J.D. and Nadel, L. (2004). Sleep, dreams, and memory consolidation: the role of the stress hormone cortisol. *Learning and Memory*;11(6):671-8.

Philip, P., Chaufton, C., Orriols, L., Lagarde, E., Amoros, E., Laumon, B., Sagaspe, P. (2014). Complaints of Poor Sleep and Risk of Traffic Accidents: A Population-Based Case-Control Study. *PLoS ONE, 9*(12), e114102.

Raudenbush, B., Koon, J., Smith, J. and Zoladz, P. (2003). Effects of odorant administration on objective and subjective measures of sleep quality, post-sleep mood and alertness, and cognitive performance. *North American Journal of Psychology;* 5(2):181-192

Sanjay R. P. and Frank B. H. (2012). Short Sleep Duration and Weight Gain: A Systematic Review. *Obesity.*

Shahrad, T., Ling, L., Diane, A., Terry, A. and Emmanuel, M. (2004). Short Sleep Duration Is Associated with Reduced Leptin, Elevated Ghrelin, and Increased Body Mass Index. *PLoS Medicine;* 1(3): e62.

Singh M., Drake CL, Roehrs T., Hudgel DW, Roth T.. The association between obesity and short sleep duration: a population-based study. *J Clin Sleep Med* 2005; **1**: 357– 363.

Sloane, P. D., Figuiero . and Cohen L. (2008). Light as Therapy for Sleep Disorders and Depression in Older Adults. *Clinical Geriatriatry;* 16(3): 25–31.

Spiegel, K., Leproult, R. and Van Cauter, E. (1999). Impact of sleep debt on metabolic and endocrine function. *Lancet;* 354(9188):1435–1439.

Stussman, B.J., Black, L.I., Barnes, P.M., Clarke, T.C., Nahin, R.L. (2012). Wellness-related use of common

181

complementary health approaches among adults: United States, 2012. National health statistics reports; no 85. Hyattsville, MD: National Center for Health Statistics.

Tsuno, N., Besset, A., & Ritchie, K. (2005). Sleep and Depression. *The Journal of Clinical Psychiatry*, *66*(10), 1254–1269.

van Leeuwen, W. M. A., Hublin, C., Sallinen, M., Härmä, M., Hirvonen, A., & Porkka-Heiskanen, T. (2010). Prolonged Sleep Restriction Affects Glucose Metabolism in Healthy Young Men. *International Journal of Endocrinology*, *2010*, 1–7.

Walker, M. P., Liston, C., Hobson, J. A., & Stickgold, R. (2002). Cognitive flexibility across the sleep–wake cycle: REM-sleep enhancement of anagram problem solving. *Cognitive Brain Research*, *14*(3), 317–324.

Wetter, D. W., & Young, T. B. (1994). The Relation Between Cigarette Smoking and Sleep Disturbance. *Preventive Medicine*, *23*(3), 328–334.

Made in the USA
Columbia, SC
20 January 2025

52149071R00109